# ScrubTales™ Physician Assistant

A Real-World Career Guide That Tells the Truth About Practicing Medicine Within a Team-Based System

ScrubTales™ Series 1 — Core Clinical Careers

Mason Preddy

MMP
MASON MAISON
PUBLISHING™
REWRITING THE NARRATIVE
MASONMAISON.PUB

MASON MAISON
PUBLISHING™
REWRITING THE NARRATIVE
MASONMAISON.PUB

**Copyright & Disclaimer**



**ScrubTales™ — Physician Assistant** is an informational and educational resource designed to support career exploration, professional reflection, and informed decision-making within healthcare. It is not intended to replace formal education, clinical training, professional judgment, legal counsel, or guidance from accredited educational programs, certifying bodies, employers, or regulatory agencies.

The information presented reflects general industry practices, lived-experience patterns, and workforce realities at the time of writing. Healthcare roles, scope of practice, licensure requirements, certification standards, compensation structures, and employment conditions vary by state, country, institution, specialty, and over time. Readers are responsible for verifying current requirements and regulations with appropriate licensing boards, accrediting organizations, educational institutions, and employers.

This book does not provide medical advice, legal advice, financial advice, or guarantees of employment, compensation, career satisfaction, or professional outcomes. Career decisions involve personal responsibility, contextual judgment, and evolving circumstances. The author and publisher make no representations or warranties regarding outcomes associated with the use of this material.

ScrubTales™ is built on the principle that alignment matters—but alignment does not remove responsibility, complexity, or accountability inherent in healthcare practice. The purpose of this book is not to persuade readers toward or away from the Physician Assistant profession, but to offer a clear-eyed view of the role as it is lived, so readers can make decisions they are prepared to stand behind.

Printed in the United States of America.

To **Todd A. Pickard, DMSc, PA-C, DFAAPA, FASCO** — President and Chair of the American Academy of Physician Associates — whose leadership bridges practice and possibility.

Your career stands as living proof that alignment isn't found in titles, but in purpose. Through decades of service, you've advanced the Physician Assistant profession from support role to strategic partner, from helper to healer, from "mid-level" to mission-critical.

Your voice reminds every PA student, educator, and clinician that excellence is not granted by hierarchy, but earned through advocacy, empathy, and evidence. In your hands, the profession doesn't just grow — it evolves.

May this dedication echo your example: that modern medicine moves forward when we all practice at the top of our compassion.

**“Practice Without Pride, Lead Without Title”**

“Physician Assistants practice without pride and lead without title, proving that mastery in medicine begins with humility and ends with healing.”

Chapter 1

# A Note to the Reader

Throughout this book, you will occasionally see a term followed by **(gl)**. This indicates that the word appears in the back-of-book glossary, where you can find a clear, reader-friendly definition. Healthcare—especially Physician Assistant practice—uses a large amount of clinical shorthand, technical terminology, and professional language that may be unfamiliar at first. The (gl) markers are included to make learning smoother, allowing you to quickly look up important concepts without interrupting your reading flow. Over time, these terms will become part of your everyday professional vocabulary.

Chapter 2
# Welcome

If you're holding this book, you're likely standing at an important crossroads—whether you're considering becoming a Physician Assistant, already on that path, or quietly questioning whether the role you're in still fits the person you are becoming.

This book exists to meet you exactly there.

**ScrubTales™ — Physician Assistant** is not a brochure for the profession, and it isn't a warning label either. It's a lived-reality system designed to help you understand what this career actually asks of you—day after day, decision after decision—so you can choose with clarity rather than momentum.

Physician Assistants occupy a unique and powerful space in healthcare. The role carries clinical responsibility, cognitive load, and relational intensity that are often underestimated from the outside. It can be deeply meaningful, intellectually engaging, and professionally rewarding. It can also be exhausting, morally complex, and structurally constrained in ways that surprise even highly capable people. Both truths can exist at the same time.

This book does not assume that ability equals fit.

You can be smart enough, driven enough, compassionate enough—and still find yourself misaligned with the realities of PA practice. That does not mean you failed. It means you deserve better information before committing years of training, debt, identity, and energy to a role that may or may not sustain you long term.

You'll notice early on that this book invites honesty. About workload. About autonomy. About supervision. About the emotional toll of decision-making and responsibility. About the difference between loving patient care and surviving healthcare systems. These conversations are often softened, delayed, or skipped entirely until people are already in too deep. That is exactly what this book is trying to prevent.

You are not expected to read this straight through.

Instead, think of this as a reference system you'll return to at different moments—before applying to school, during training, while interviewing, or years into practice when something starts to feel off. The structure is intentional. Each section is designed to stand on its own while also revealing patterns when viewed together.

Above all, this book respects your agency.

It will not tell you who you should be. It will not promise ease, prestige, or fulfillment. What it offers is something more durable: a way to evaluate fit honestly, before the cost of course-correcting becomes too high.

If this book helps you move forward with confidence, pause with clarity, or choose a different path entirely—then it has done its job.

Welcome to ScrubTales™.

Chapter 3

# How to Use This Book

This book is not designed to be consumed in order—and it's not meant to be finished in a single pass. **ScrubTales™ — Physician Assistant** is built as a decision-support system, not a narrative you rush through and set aside.

You are encouraged to move through it strategically.

Some readers begin here, at the front, wanting context before committing to anything else. Others jump straight to the Day-in-the-Life Dispatches, searching for a felt sense of the work. Some land in the Financial Landscape™, the Fit Analyzer, or the Pivot Playbook because those questions feel urgent right now. All of those entry points are valid. The structure is intentional so you can return to different sections as your situation changes.

Each major component answers a different kind of question.

Some sections help you understand the *emotional and cognitive cost* of the role. Others focus on *practical realities*—education, hiring, compensation, and long-term flexibility.

Some are reflective by design, meant to slow you down rather than push you forward. Read them when you are calm, not when you are panicked or chasing a deadline.

You do not need to agree with everything in this book for it to be useful.

What matters more is noticing your reactions. Pay attention to what energizes you, what tightens your chest, what you skim past, and what you reread. Those signals often tell you more about fit than any checklist or external advice ever will.

If you are early in your journey, use this book to pressure-test your assumptions before you invest time, money, and identity into the role. If you are already in PA school or practice, use it as a mirror—one that helps you name what's working, what isn't, and what options actually exist beyond "push through" or "quit entirely."

You may also find that this book works best in stages.

Read a section. Step away. Live a little. Come back with new questions. The goal is not certainty on day one. The goal is alignment over time—making choices you understand, accept, and are prepared to stand behind.

There is no single correct way to use this book.

There is only the way that helps you make a decision you can live with.

Chapter 4

# Why This Book Exists

This book exists because too many people are making one of the most consequential decisions of their lives with incomplete information—and then blaming themselves when the reality doesn't match the promise.

The Physician Assistant role is often presented as a smart compromise: meaningful clinical work, strong job demand, flexibility across specialties, and a more balanced alternative to other clinical paths. For some people, that description holds true. For others, it obscures the parts of the role that matter most once the novelty wears off—pace, supervision dynamics, cognitive burden, emotional responsibility, and the systems that quietly shape how the work actually feels.

Most resources focus on *whether you can become* a PA.

This book is focused on whether you should—given who you are, how you're wired, what you need to thrive, and what you're willing to carry long term.

Over the years, I've watched highly capable, deeply committed people enter healthcare roles they were technically suited for but structurally misaligned with. They didn't struggle because they lacked intelligence or grit. They struggled because the day-to-day realities of the job conflicted with their identity, values, energy patterns, or tolerance for ambiguity and constraint. By the time that truth surfaced, the cost of course-correcting was already high.

The Physician Assistant profession deserves better conversations than that.

So do the people considering it.

This book exists to surface the conversations that are usually postponed until burnout, resentment, or quiet dissatisfaction forces them into the open. It talks plainly about responsibility without autonomy, about caring deeply inside systems that often reward speed over presence, and about the difference between enjoying medicine and surviving healthcare.

It also exists to honor the many Physician Assistants who *are* aligned—who find meaning, sustainability, and pride in the work they do. Their experiences matter too. Alignment is not rare, but it is specific. What works beautifully for one person may slowly erode another.

This book does not argue for or against the PA profession.

It argues for informed choice.

If you decide this path fits you, you should enter it with your eyes open and your expectations grounded in reality. If you decide it doesn't, that decision deserves respect—not shame, not justification, not silence.

This book exists so fewer people have to learn these lessons the hard way.

Chapter 5

# Who This Book Is For (and Who It Isn't)

This book is for people who want to make a deliberate decision—not a rushed one, not a borrowed one, and not a decision driven by momentum or outside pressure.

It is for those considering the Physician Assistant profession who want to understand what the work actually asks of them beyond prerequisites, acceptance letters, and job descriptions. It's for students who are already in PA school and beginning to sense the weight of responsibility, pace, and expectation that accompanies the role. And it's for practicing Physician Assistants who may be quietly reassessing fit, sustainability, or long-term direction—even if they're good at what they do.

This book is for people who value honesty over reassurance.

It's for readers willing to look at tradeoffs without flinching, to name both the privilege and the pressure of clinical decision-making, and to acknowledge that professional success and personal alignment are not always the same thing. It's for those who want language for what they're feeling but haven't been able to articulate—and for those who want permission to ask harder questions before committing further.

This book is also for people who understand that alignment is not about ease.

The Physician Assistant role carries real responsibility, cognitive load, and accountability. If you are drawn to meaningful work and are prepared to shoulder that weight thoughtfully, this book will help you evaluate whether the structure of PA practice supports you—or slowly works against you.

This book is **not** for people looking for guarantees.

It is not a shortcut to certainty, a promise of work-life balance, or a reassurance that everything will work out if you just try hard enough. It is not written to sell the profession, justify past decisions, or soften uncomfortable realities. If you are seeking affirmation without examination, this book may feel challenging.

It is also not for those who want a single "right answer."

Healthcare careers are complex, context-dependent, and deeply personal. This book does not replace mentorship, lived experience, or professional judgment. What it offers instead is a framework for thinking clearly—so the choice you make is one you understand and can stand behind.

If you are ready for that kind of honesty, this book is for you.

If not, that's okay too. Timing matters.

Chapter 6

# Note on Alignment, Responsibility, and Choice

Alignment is often misunderstood as comfort, ease, or constant satisfaction. In healthcare—especially in roles with clinical responsibility—alignment is something quieter and more demanding than that.

Alignment means the work you do matches who you are, how you're wired, and what you need to sustain effort over time. It does not remove pressure. It does not eliminate difficult days, complex patients, or emotionally heavy decisions. What it does is reduce the internal friction that occurs when a role consistently asks you to operate against your nature, values, or limits.

The Physician Assistant role carries real responsibility.

Clinical judgment, decision-making under uncertainty, managing risk, navigating supervision structures, and advocating for patients within imperfect systems are not abstract concepts—they are daily realities. Alignment does not make these responsibilities lighter, but it can make them feel *worth carrying.*

This book asks you to take responsibility seriously.

Not just responsibility to patients, but responsibility to yourself. To understand the tradeoffs you are accepting. To recognize the difference between temporary discomfort and chronic misalignment. To acknowledge that choosing a role is also choosing a set of constraints, expectations, and long-term demands—many of which will shape your life outside of work as much as inside it.

Choice is central here.

You may not control every variable in healthcare, but you do control how intentionally you enter it. Choosing this profession with open eyes is an act of respect—for yourself, for the patients you will serve, and for the people who will depend on your decisions.

This book does not frame alignment as destiny.

It frames it as an ongoing relationship between you and your work—one that evolves as your life, values, and circumstances change. Alignment today does not guarantee alignment forever. What matters is building the skill of noticing when fit shifts and responding with clarity rather than denial.

As you move through this book, you will be invited to reflect—not just on whether you *can* do this work, but on whether you want to do it under the conditions that actually exist.

That question is not selfish.

It is responsible.

Chapter 7

# Introduction to the SCRUBfits™ — Meet the SCRUBfits™

Before you dive into the realities of the Physician Assistant role, you'll be introduced to a set of guides you'll encounter throughout this book: the **SCRUB*fits*™**.

The **SCRUB*fits*™** are not mascots, stereotypes, or personality labels. They are alignment archetypes—ways of noticing how different people experience the same work very differently depending on who they are, how they're wired, and what they need to thrive. Think of them as mirrors, not categories you're supposed to fit into.

Each **SCRUB*fit*™** represents a pattern of motivation, tolerance, energy, and fulfillment that shows up again and again across healthcare careers. None of them are better than the others. None of them are "right." What matters is recognizing which ones feel familiar to you—and which ones don't.

As you move through the Day-in-the-Life Dispatches, the Toll Booth, decision points, and reflection sections, you'll see the

**SCRUB*fits*™** referenced as interpretive anchors. They help surface questions like:

Who tends to feel energized by this moment?

Who might quietly struggle here over time?

What kind of person thrives under these conditions—and why?

You may see yourself clearly in one **SCRUB*fit*™**. You may recognize pieces of yourself in several. You may notice that a **SCRUB*fit*™** you once identified with no longer fits as your life has changed. All of that is normal.

The purpose of the **SCRUB*fits*™** is not to predict your future or box you into an identity.

Their purpose is to help you notice patterns—especially the subtle ones that often get missed when decisions are made under pressure or excitement. They give language to experiences that are otherwise dismissed as "just part of the job," even when those experiences are slowly draining or misaligned.

As you read, pay attention to your reactions.

When a **SCRUB*fit*™** feels uncomfortably accurate, pause. When one feels completely foreign, notice that too. These responses are not judgments—they are data. And data, when taken seriously, protects you from costly assumptions.

The **SCRUB*fits*™** will walk with you throughout this book, not to lead you to a conclusion, but to help you arrive at one you can stand behind.

Chapter 8

# PACES™ and CARESET™ in Physician Assistant Practice —

**PACES™ & CARESET™** *in Physician Assistant Practice — Why This Career Fits Some People Beautifully — and Breaks Others Quietly*

Physician Assistant practice sits at a powerful intersection of medicine, responsibility, and relational care. It is clinically demanding, cognitively rigorous, and emotionally intimate. For some, it feels like the precise expression of their professional identity. For others, it becomes a quiet grind they struggle to explain. The difference is rarely intelligence, work ethic, or training.

The difference is alignment.

In **Mason's Alignment Theory (MAT)**, alignment is not accidental, nor is it abstract. It emerges from the interaction between two lenses: **PACES™**, which reflects the internal drivers shaping how you experience work, and **CARESET™**, which reflects the external conditions shaping how the work is structured around you.

**PACES™** represents the five internal forces that determine how a role feels from the inside:

**P — Personality**

**A — Aptitude**

**C — Constraints**

**E — Experience**

**S — Situation**

These elements influence not whether you can perform the work, but whether you can sustain it without eroding yourself.

**CARESET™** represents the seven external conditions that determine how the professional environment interacts with you:

**C — Culture**

**A — Autonomy**

**R — Resources**

**E — Expectations**

**S — Structure**

**E — Environment**

**T — Team**

These conditions shape whether the role reinforces or strains your internal wiring.

In Physician Assistant practice, both lenses matter deeply because the role is elastic. It expands or contracts based on setting, supervising physician style, patient population, institutional culture, and life stage. The title "Physician Assistant" tells you very little about how the job will actually feel.

Through **PACES™**, we begin internally.

**Personality** influences how you metabolize pace and pressure. Some PAs are energized by high-acuity environments where rapid decision-making and constant collaboration are the norm. Emergency departments, surgical services, and inpatient specialties can feel alive and purposeful to them. Others are steadied by longitudinal care, predictable clinic rhythms, and deeper patient relationships built over time. Primary care, outpatient specialties, or subspecialty follow-up clinics may offer a more sustainable cadence. Neither personality profile is superior. Misalignment appears when your nervous system is forced into a tempo it was not built to maintain.

**Aptitude** reflects your capacity to synthesize data, tolerate uncertainty, and manage layered responsibility. PA education builds technical competence across disciplines, but aptitude also includes how comfortably you hold ambiguity. Medicine rarely offers perfect clarity. If uncertainty consistently unsettles you, high-complexity specialties may feel draining rather than stimulating. Conversely, if you require intellectual challenge to feel engaged, highly protocol-driven settings may feel stifling. The technical demands of the role are teachable; how those demands land internally is not.

**Constraints** operate quietly but powerfully. Educational debt, geographic limitations, family responsibilities, caregiving roles, and financial obligations narrow the range of choices available. A PA who must remain in a specific region may accept a role misaligned with personality or long-term goals. A parent balancing young children may choose predictability over prestige. Constraints do not indicate weakness; they reflect reality. However, when constraints force prolonged misalignment, resentment can accumulate beneath professionalism.

**Experience** changes how the role feels over time. The first year of practice often brings adrenaline and growth. By year five or ten, repetition may replace novelty. What once felt exhilarating may begin to feel relentless. Alternatively, increased mastery may create deeper satisfaction and confidence. Experience modifies the emotional weight of the same responsibilities. A sustainable PA career requires recalibration as experience evolves.

**Situation** captures timing. Season of life matters. Entering PA practice at twenty-five feels different than entering at forty-five. Health changes, family shifts, economic climates, and institutional restructuring alter how manageable the same workload feels. A role that fits beautifully during one season may feel misaligned during another. Recognizing situational shifts prevents self-blame when the internal landscape changes.

If **PACES™** explains how you experience the role, **CARESET™** explains how the role experiences you.

**Culture** defines the emotional climate of a practice. In some environments, questions are welcomed, mistakes are framed as learning opportunities, and collaboration feels genuine. In others, hierarchy dominates, feedback is punitive, and silence becomes self-protection. A supportive culture amplifies confidence; a corrosive culture drains it.

**Autonomy** is central to PA satisfaction. The profession was built on collaborative practice, yet the degree of independence varies widely. Some PAs are trusted to evaluate, diagnose, and manage patients with significant discretion. Others function under restrictive oversight, limited decision-making authority, or inconsistent supervisory support. Too little autonomy can feel infantilizing. Too much autonomy without support can feel perilous. The balance determines whether responsibility feels empowering or destabilizing.

**Resources** determine whether you can practice safely and efficiently. Adequate staffing, access to diagnostic tools, administrative support, reasonable patient volumes, and functional technology systems protect professional stamina. Resource scarcity transforms routine care into chronic strain. Even highly resilient PAs fatigue when asked to compensate continuously for systemic gaps.

**Expectations** define what "enough" means. How many patients are reasonable? How are mistakes handled? Are boundaries respected? Unclear or shifting expectations create invisible tension that accumulates over time.

**Structure** shapes workflow and predictability. Clear protocols, defined scopes of practice, transparent performance metrics, and realistic productivity targets reduce friction. Ambiguous supervision models or inconsistent accountability increase cognitive strain.

**Environment** encompasses the physical and operational setting. Inpatient floors, operating rooms, urgent care centers, and telehealth platforms each carry different sensory and logistical demands. Lighting, noise, pace, and spatial design influence energy more than many clinicians initially recognize. An environment that aligns with your stimulation threshold sustains you; one that overwhelms it erodes focus and patience.

**Team** may be the most protective factor of all. Trust, communication, and mutual respect transform heavy workloads into shared burdens. Conversely, fragmented teams amplify isolation. The PA role exists within interprofessional dynamics; when team cohesion is strong, confidence grows. When it fractures, even skilled clinicians begin to question themselves.

When **PACES™** and **CARESET™** align, PA practice feels challenging without being crushing. Responsibility feels meaningful rather than suffocating. Collaboration feels energizing rather than political. The work stretches you but does not distort you. You return home tired but intact.

When they do not align, misalignment often disguises itself as burnout. You may assume you are insufficiently resilient or insufficiently grateful. Yet the deeper issue is structural and internal mismatch — your **PACES™** profile operating within **CARESET™** conditions that amplify friction rather than reinforce fit. Over time, this produces a quiet erosion: cynicism, emotional numbing, or chronic fatigue that no vacation resolves.

The purpose of this chapter is not to declare Physician Assistant practice inherently good or bad. It is to illuminate the architecture beneath the experience.

Two PAs in the same specialty, within the same hospital, can report radically different levels of satisfaction because their internal drivers and external conditions interact differently.

Before commitment turns into momentum, pause. Consider how your **PACES™** profile intersects with the **CARESET™** realities of the setting you are entering. Ask how decisions are made. Ask how autonomy is structured. Ask how support appears during complications. Ask how productivity is measured. Reflect on your constraints and your current season of life. Examine whether you are seeking stimulation, stability, growth, or recalibration.

Alignment is not about perfection.

It is about fit.

In Physician Assistant practice, fit determines whether the role becomes a sustainable professional home or a position you endure while quietly planning your exit.

When you understand this early — through the lens of **Mason's Alignment Theory (MAT)** — you protect more than your career. You protect your energy, your relationships, and your long-term professional identity.

That is the real work of alignment.

## Chapter 9
# The Toll Booth –

***The Emotional, Cognitive, and Lifestyle Cost of Being a Physician Assistant***

Every career has a cost.

Not the kind you see on a tuition bill or a loan statement – but the quieter cost that accumulates slowly, paid in attention, energy, and emotional bandwidth. The toll you don't notice at first because it's charged in small increments, one shift at a time.

For Physician Assistants, that toll is rarely collected all at once.

It shows up in the constant mental readiness – the need to stay sharp, alert, and accountable even when you're tired. It lives in the handoff moments, the chart you replay in your head on the drive home, the patient encounter that lingers longer than it should. It's the responsibility of knowing that your decisions matter, even when they're made under time pressure, incomplete information, or competing priorities.

This is not a criticism of the role.

It's a description of it.

PA practice sits in a unique space. You are trained to act with clinical judgment, yet you practice within layers of supervision, policy, and organizational expectation. Some days that balance feels collaborative and supportive. Other days it feels constraining — especially when responsibility outpaces authority, or when you're expected to move quickly without the structural backing to do so safely.

The emotional toll often arrives quietly.

You may find yourself absorbing patients' fear, frustration, and grief — then setting it aside to move on to the next room. You may become skilled at compartmentalizing, only to realize later that the compartments are filling faster than they empty. The work requires presence, empathy, and professionalism, even on days when your own reserves are thin.

Cognitively, the load is relentless.

Clinical reasoning doesn't end when the shift does. Differential diagnoses echo. "What ifs" surface at inconvenient moments. The responsibility to stay current — guidelines, protocols, evolving evidence — is ongoing, not optional. Even in supportive environments, the mental hum of the role rarely goes fully quiet.

And then there's the lifestyle cost.

Schedules that look manageable on paper can feel very different in practice. Early mornings, late evenings, rotating shifts, call expectations, documentation that spills into personal time. Flexibility exists in some PA roles — but it's unevenly distributed, and often traded for other pressures. What gives you autonomy in one area may demand availability in another.

None of this means the toll is unbearable.

For many Physician Assistants, it's worth it. The work aligns with who they are. The responsibility feels meaningful rather than heavy. The tradeoffs make sense within the context of their values, season of life, and support systems.

The problem arises when the toll is paid without acknowledgment.

When you believe discomfort means weakness.

When you assume everyone else is handling it better than you are.

When you keep pushing because you're capable — not because you're aligned.

This is the first checkpoint.

Not to scare you.

Not to discourage you.

But to ask a necessary question early, before the toll becomes invisible:

*Am I willing — and equipped — to pay this cost, not just for a year or two, but over time?*

There is no right answer.

Only an honest one.

And honesty, here, is not a liability.

It's protection.

## Chapter 10

# Day-in-the-Life Dispatches —

***Twelve Windows Into the Lived Reality of PA Practice***

Job descriptions flatten reality.

They list responsibilities, settings, and scope of practice, but they rarely capture how the work *actually feels* once you're inside it — the rhythm of a day, the moments that energize you, the ones that quietly drain you, and the cumulative effect of carrying responsibility across hours, weeks, and years.

These dispatches exist to restore that missing dimension.

Each Day-in-the-Life is a window into a real working day as a Physician Assistant — not an idealized version, not a worst-case scenario, but a lived one. You'll move through mornings and handoffs, patient encounters and documentation, collaboration and constraint. You'll hear internal dialogue most professionals don't say out loud. You'll notice how the pace lands, how decisions are made, and what lingers when the shift ends.

Some days will feel familiar immediately.

Others may surprise you.

A few may unsettle you in ways you can't quite name.

That response matters.

These dispatches are not meant to convince you that PA practice is right for you — or wrong. They are meant to help you notice patterns. Where your attention sharpens. Where your shoulders tense. Where you feel pulled forward versus quietly resistant.

Read them slowly. Not all at once.

Return to them after other chapters.

Notice which ones stay with you.

The goal here isn't to imagine whether you *could* do this work.

It's to ask a more durable question:

*What would it be like to live inside this role — day after day — and does that life align with who I am, how I'm wired, and what I need to thrive?*

The answers won't arrive all at once.

But they will begin to take shape.

—

***Day-in-the-Life Dispatch #1 —***

***Primary Care: The Long View***

The day starts before the first patient arrives.

Not officially — the schedule doesn't reflect it — but practically. Charts are reviewed, labs scanned, messages triaged. There's a quiet mental sorting that happens as you sip coffee and log in, already anticipating which visits will be straightforward and which will require more time than the template allows.

Primary care is built on continuity, but continuity carries weight.

By mid-morning, you've already shifted gears half a dozen times. A routine follow-up turns into a conversation about housing insecurity. A medication refill opens the door to unmanaged anxiety. Preventive care lives side by side with problems no guideline fully addresses.

You listen. You redirect. You document — constantly aware of the clock, but equally aware that rushing the wrong moment can cost trust you've spent years building.

Between patients, messages accumulate. Results need explanation. Referrals need justification. Prior authorizations quietly consume attention they never seem to earn. You practice medicine in the spaces between screens, doing your best to stay present while navigating systems that rarely slow down to match the complexity of real lives.

The autonomy is real here — but so is the responsibility.

You are often the steady point. The familiar face. The one patients return to when symptoms blur together or when life circumstances complicate medical plans. That trust is meaningful. It's also heavy. You carry stories forward, even when the day moves on.

By late afternoon, cognitive fatigue sets in. Not from crisis, but from accumulation. Decision after decision. Small judgments that add up. You finish notes where you can, knowing some will follow you home.

When the last patient leaves, the work doesn't fully end.

There's satisfaction — in relationships built, in care coordinated, in being the person someone turns to when things feel unclear. There's also a quiet question that surfaces as you shut down your computer:

*Can I carry this pace, this responsibility, this kind of presence — sustainably — over time?*

For some Physician Assistants, the answer is yes. The long view fits. The continuity nourishes rather than drains.

For others, this setting reveals a mismatch — not of skill, but of energy and need.

Notice your reaction here.

That reaction is information.

Chapter 11

# Day In The Life -- Family Medicine / Primary Care

**04:47 a.m.**

The alarm goes off once. Avery Maddox, PA-C doesn't hit snooze. Family medicine days don't allow for that kind of optimism. Avery swings their legs out of bed before the sound fully dies, feet hitting the cold hardwood like a starter pistol.

Ranger is already awake. Golden retriever. Eighty pounds. Too smart for his own good. His tail thumps against the wall in steady approval: *Yes. Good. This is correct. We are awake.*

Juniper, the black cat, does not move. She opens one eye, judges the situation, and closes it again.

Avery pads into the kitchen, starts the coffee, and cracks two eggs into a pan. Real breakfast today. Family medicine requires fuel. Scrambled eggs, sourdough toast, half an avocado with salt and red pepper flakes. Avery eats standing up at the counter, scrolling the clinic schedule on their phone.

Twenty-six patients booked. Three same-day slots. No breathing room.

On the fridge, a magnet holds yesterday's lab reminder. Avery snaps a picture of it. That patient's A1C was trending the wrong direction. They'll need a hard conversation today.

**05:36 a.m.**

Scrubs on. Badge clipped. Stethoscope in the bag. Avery checks the mirror—neutral face, hair pulled back, no visible fatigue. Ranger gets fed. Juniper gets fed something that costs more than Avery's breakfast and acts like it's beneath her.

Keys. Wallet. Phone.

**05:52 a.m.**

The drive in is quiet. Avery drives an aging SUV that smells faintly like dog and hand sanitizer. Sunrise hasn't started yet, just a pale line cutting the horizon. No podcast. No music. Avery runs through the day mentally—who needs close supervision, who can move fast, who is going to take time whether the schedule allows it or not.

**06:31 a.m.**

Clinic parking lot. Lights already on. Avery sits in the car for exactly ten seconds, then opens the door. Once inside, the day belongs to other people.

**06:39 a.m.**

Inbox first. Always.

Lab results. Refill requests. A patient message marked *urgent*. Avery opens it: dizziness, black stools, started a new blood thinner last week.

That gets flagged immediately.

Avery walks down the hall to the physician workroom.

Dr. Patel, MD—supervising physician—is already charting, coffee untouched.

“Morning,” Avery says.

Dr. Patel looks up. “What’s up?”

“Possible GI bleed. On anticoagulation. I’m calling him now but I think he needs ED evaluation.”

Dr. Patel nods without hesitation. “Agreed. Send him. I’ll cosign.”

That’s the relationship. No ceremony. Thirty seconds. The responsibility still sits with Avery.

**07:02 a.m.**

Phone call confirmed. Patient resistant at first. Avery explains risk clearly, calmly. No drama. Just facts. The patient agrees.

Decision one: done.

**08:00 a.m.**

First patient: annual physical. Straightforward until it isn’t. Blood pressure (gl) is high. Avery rechecks manually. Still high.

“Has anyone ever talked to you about hypertension (gl)?” Avery asks.

The patient shrugs. “They mentioned it once.”

Avery doesn’t shrug back. Medication discussion. Lifestyle questions. Family history. Labs ordered. Follow-up scheduled. Another invisible prevention moment that never makes headlines.

**08:47 a.m.**

Chest tightness. Thirty-nine years old. “Probably anxiety.”

Avery doesn’t buy “probably.”

History. Exam. EKG (gl). Normal, but the story feels wrong. Avery steps into the hall, catches Dr. Patel between rooms.

“Mind if I run this by you?” Avery asks, already summarizing.

Dr. Patel listens. “Yeah. I don’t love it either. Send them out.”

“Thanks.”

No ego. No hierarchy drama. Just shared risk.

**09:58 a.m.**

Walk-in: feverish toddler, parent exhausted and near tears. Otitis media (gl). Antibiotics. Weight-based dosing. Avery kneels to the child’s eye level, lets them hold the stethoscope. The kid stops crying. The parent exhales.

**11:14 a.m.**

Diabetes follow-up. The A1C Avery photographed this morning is worse.

Avery closes the chart and looks at the patient. “Help me understand what’s hard.”

Silence. Then the truth: strips are expensive. Food choices are limited. Work hours are brutal.

Avery adjusts medication, orders alternatives, documents carefully. This isn't noncompliance. It's systems failure.

**12:02 p.m.**

Lunch exists on the schedule. Reality disagrees.

Protein bar. Half of it. Standing. Between notes.

**12:41 p.m.**

Laceration (gl). Hand. Worksite injury. Avery assesses tendon function, sensation, circulation. Cleans, numbs, sutures (gl). The patient watches closely.

"You a doctor?" he asks.

"I'm a PA," Avery says, without defensiveness. "I do this a lot."

**01:58 p.m.**

Teen visit. Stomach pain. Mother answering too fast.

Avery asks the mother to step out.

The truth comes quietly. Mental health. Safety concerns. Avery listens, asks the right questions, loops Dr. Patel in briefly. Plan formed. Resources given. Follow-up arranged.

This is family medicine too.

**03:36 p.m.**

Another walk-in. Another blood pressure crisis. Avery manages, adjusts, documents. The mental load stacks invisibly.

**04:49 p.m.**

Last patient leaves. The clinic quiets. Avery does not.

Notes. Orders. Results. Messages.

**05:32 p.m.**

Dr. Patel passes by. “Good work today.”

Avery nods. It helps. It doesn’t erase the fatigue.

**06:07 p.m.**

Drive home. No music. Just the road and the hum of exhaustion that isn’t burnout yet—but knows how to get there.

**06:41 p.m.**

Home. Ranger explodes with joy. Juniper pretends Avery never left.

Dinner is rotisserie chicken and salad. Functional. Shared with a partner who listens, but doesn’t press for details. Some days don’t translate.

**09:18 p.m.**

Scrubs in the hamper. Tomorrow’s set folded.

Avery sets the alarm.

In the dark, the thought surfaces—not dramatic, just honest:

*I did good work today. The question is how many days like this fit into a life.*

The alarm is already waiting.

Chapter 12

# Day In The Life -- Urgent Care

**06:12 a.m.**

The alarm goes off later on urgent care days, but the trade-off is brutal honesty: the schedule may look lighter, but nothing about it is predictable.

Jordan Reyes, PA-C rolls onto their side and shuts the alarm off before it wakes the rest of the house. Today is a **12-hour urgent care shift** — open to close. No call. No rounding. Just a steady stream of whatever walks through the door.

Biscuit, a squat, snoring English bulldog, lifts his head long enough to confirm that Jordan is, in fact, awake, then collapses again like gravity has increased. Luna, the gray tabby cat, uses the moment to step directly onto Jordan's chest as if this were always the plan.

"Okay," Jordan mutters. "I'm up."

**06:24 a.m.**

Coffee goes on first. Breakfast is utilitarian: Greek yogurt, a banana, and a handful of almonds eaten at the counter while scrolling the urgent care staffing group chat. Someone called out. Of course they did.

Jordan is a **Physician Assistant in Urgent Care**, three years out of training. High autonomy. Broad scope. Physician supervision is remote but available — until it isn't.

Scrubs. Hair back. Badge clipped. No stethoscope today — it lives at the clinic. Less weight to carry, more responsibility instead.

**06:58 a.m.**

The drive is short. Seven minutes if the lights cooperate. Jordan listens to nothing. The brain needs to stay loose.

**07:06 a.m.**

The clinic door opens. The smell hits first: disinfectant, old coffee, faint panic.

Dr. Nguyen, DO — supervising physician — is already logged in from home. Jordan sees the green dot next to his name in the system. That dot matters more than most people realize.

**07:15 a.m.**

First patient is already waiting. The sign says *urgent care*, not *convenient care*, but expectations never read the sign.

Ankle injury. Basketball. Swelling obvious. Jordan examines, orders X-rays (gl), confirms a distal fibula fracture (gl). Explains the plan. Boot. Crutches. Orthopedic follow-up. The patient nods, relieved that someone took it seriously.

**08:02 a.m.**

Upper respiratory symptoms. "Just wants antibiotics."

Jordan doesn't budge. Viral. No pneumonia signs. Education instead of a prescription. The patient leaves annoyed. Jordan documents carefully. Urgent care requires defensible restraint as much as intervention.

**08:41 a.m.**

Chest pain. Again. Different kind.

Jordan pauses. This isn't primary care. There's no luxury of long evaluation. Jordan runs the protocol: vitals, EKG (gl), history sharp and fast. The EKG isn't normal.

Jordan messages Dr. Nguyen immediately.

**Jordan:** "EKG w/ ST changes. 54yo male. Sending to ED."

**Dr. Nguyen:** "Agree. Call EMS. I'll cosign."

Thirty seconds. The decision sticks to Jordan's ribs like pressure.

**09:27 a.m.**

Laceration (gl). Kitchen knife. Jordan irrigates, anesthetizes, sutures (gl). The patient watches closely.

"You a doctor?"

"I'm a PA," Jordan says. "This is what I do."

The answer is practiced. Neutral. True.

**10:18 a.m.**

Burn. Second degree (gl). Grill accident. Jordan cools, cleans, dresses the wound, reviews signs of infection. Pain management discussion. The patient is grateful. Gratitude helps — briefly.

**11:06 a.m.**

A child with fever and a parent who is terrified of meningitis (gl). Jordan examines carefully, reassures honestly, gives strict return precautions. The parent relaxes just enough to breathe.

**12:01 p.m.**

Lunch is technically allowed. Practically, it's a protein shake behind the desk while reviewing radiology reports.

**12:37 p.m.**

Back-to-back. Sprain. UTI (gl). Rash. Someone angry about wait times. Someone crying because they don't have insurance and don't know where else to go.

Urgent care sees the overflow of the system — and absorbs the frustration.

**02:04 p.m.**

Shortness of breath. Jordan doesn't like the way this one looks. Oxygen saturation (gl) borderline. History concerning.

Jordan calls Dr. Nguyen.

"Can you look at this with me?"

Dr. Nguyen joins the chart, reviews, agrees. ED transfer again.

Two transfers in one shift. The day tightens.

**03:19 p.m.**

Head injury. No loss of consciousness. Nausea present. Jordan runs concussion protocol (gl), educates carefully. The patient is young, scared, trying not to show it.

**04:42 p.m.**

Foot pain that turns out to be cellulitis (gl). Antibiotics. Clear instructions. Jordan emphasizes return signs. Urgent care is often the first — and last — line before something worsens.

**05:58 p.m.**

The waiting room is still full. Energy is low. Focus is high. Jordan's shoulders ache. The pace never let up.

**07:11 p.m.**

Last patient leaves. The clinic finally exhales.

Jordan signs charts, clears messages, checks that Dr. Nguyen has cosigned everything requiring it. That green dot is still there.

**07:34 p.m.**

Drive home. Exhaustion hits like delayed onset. The kind that waits politely until you're safe to feel it.

**07:45 p.m.**

Home. Biscuit greets Jordan like they've returned from war. Luna pretends nothing happened.

Dinner is reheated leftovers. Quiet. Phone face-down. The day doesn't get to follow Jordan into the evening.

**10:02 p.m.**

Shower. Bed. Muscles heavy.

Urgent care days don't linger emotionally the way others do — but they leave a residue. Decisions made fast. Risks assessed in compressed time.

In the dark, Jordan thinks:

*I handled what walked in today. The question is what keeps walking in — and how long I want to be the one standing here.*

The alarm is off tomorrow.

Chapter 13

# Day In The Life -- Emergency Medicine

**05:01 a.m.**

The alarm goes off hard because emergency medicine doesn't allow gentle mornings. Sam Carter, PA-C opens one eye, then both, already running the shift in their head. Twelve hours. Level II trauma center. Nights bleed into days here in ways the body never quite forgives.

Moose, a seventy-pound mutt with a blocky head and zero sense of personal space, is already standing on Sam's chest like a sentry. No cat today. Just Moose, breathing directly into Sam's face.

"Alright," Sam says. "I'm up."

**05:12 a.m.**

Coffee. Two cups. Breakfast is peanut butter toast and a banana eaten fast, standing, phone propped against the backsplash with overnight ED messages already lighting it up.

Sam works **Emergency Medicine** full time, four years in, comfortable but never casual.

Scrubs are darker today. Blood shows less.

**05:46 a.m.**

Drive in. City still half asleep. Ambulance sirens cut through the quiet like punctuation marks. Sam doesn't listen to music — the brain needs bandwidth.

**06:14 a.m.**

Badge swipe. The ED smells like antiseptic, stale coffee, and adrenaline. Whiteboard already full.

Dr. Klein, MD — attending physician — is mid-sign-out, coffee in hand, eyes sharp. Sam grabs a spot at the workstation.

"Beds are stacked," Dr. Klein says without preamble. "Trauma came in at 3. Psych boarding again. You're in Fast Track and flexing to main when needed."

Sam nods. That's the assignment.

**06:29 a.m.**

First patient: chest pain. Again. It always starts there.

Sam moves fast — history, vitals, EKG (gl). Looks borderline. Sam doesn't hesitate.

"Room him in main," Sam tells the nurse. "I want labs and a repeat EKG."

Sam catches Dr. Klein immediately.

"Can you eyeball this with me?"

Dr. Klein scans the strip. “Good catch. I’ll take it.”

That’s emergency medicine: seconds matter, ego doesn’t.

**07:11 a.m.**

Fast Track fills instantly. Ankle injury. Facial laceration (gl). Flu symptoms. Sam bounces between rooms, switching cognitive gears with muscle memory.

Laceration repair means focus — irrigation, local anesthetic, sutures (gl). The patient winces.

“You a doctor?”

“I’m a PA,” Sam says. “You’re in good hands.”

It’s not reassurance. It’s fact.

**08:04 a.m.**

EMS rolls in unannounced. Elderly patient. Altered mental status (gl). Unknown baseline.

Sam moves with the team — IV access, labs, CT ordered. Sam briefs Dr. Klein fast and clean.

“I think this is sepsis (gl). BP’s soft. Lactate’s coming.”

Dr. Klein nods. “Start fluids. Broad-spectrum antibiotics. I’ll be in.”

The weight lands immediately. Emergency medicine doesn’t give you time to feel it first.

**09:27 a.m.**

A young adult with abdominal pain that doesn’t make sense. Sam digs. Subtle guarding. Pain out of proportion.

Sam pauses. Reassesses. Orders imaging.

Appendicitis (gl). Early, but real.

Sam updates Dr. Klein.

“Agree,” he says. “Call surgery.”

Sam makes the call.

**10:43 a.m.**

Psych patient. Agitated. Verbal escalation. Security nearby. Sam keeps voice low, body angled, hands visible. De-escalation is a skill they don’t teach enough of.

The patient eventually sits. Breathing slows.

Sam feels the adrenaline drain late — the way it always does.

**12:02 p.m.**

Lunch is theoretical. Sam drinks a protein shake while charting, eyes flicking up every time the overhead speaker crackles.

**12:38 p.m.**

Trauma alert.

Sam moves to the bay automatically. Roles clear. Airway secure. IVs placed. Blood everywhere. Time compresses.

Sam manages procedures they’ve done hundreds of times and still respect deeply. No room for hesitation. No room for mistakes.

Dr. Klein calls the shots. Sam executes.

**02:17 p.m.**

The trauma goes upstairs. The room empties. Sam finally exhales.

Hands shake slightly. Sam notices. Lets it pass.

**03:06 p.m.**

Fast Track again. Sore throats. UTIs (gl). A patient furious about wait times.

Sam absorbs it. Documents carefully. Emergency medicine teaches you how to carry other people's anger without letting it root.

**04:29 p.m.**

Shortness of breath. Oxygen saturation (gl) dropping. Sam escalates quickly. Nebulizers. Steroids. Calls respiratory therapy.

Dr. Klein checks in.

"You good?"

"Yeah," Sam says. "This one's turning."

Dr. Klein stays close anyway.

**05:58 p.m.**

Boarded patients line the hallways. No beds upstairs. The ED becomes a holding zone for the system's failures.

Sam answers questions families shouldn't have to ask here.

**06:47 p.m.**

Last hour drags. Mental fatigue sets in. Sam double-checks everything now. That's when mistakes happen — when you assume.

**07:13 p.m.**

Sign-out. Clean. Thorough. Sam hands off each patient like they matter — because they do.

Dr. Klein claps Sam on the shoulder. "Solid shift."

It lands.

**07:29 p.m.**

Locker room. Scrubs off. Hands washed longer than necessary. The day rinses off in layers.

**07:52 p.m.**

Drive home. Sirens still echo in Sam's head even when the road is quiet.

**08:11 p.m.**

Home. Moose greets Sam like the apocalypse has been averted. Sam sinks onto the floor, face buried in fur, grounding hard.

Dinner is whatever's easy. The TV stays off. Noise feels wrong.

**10:04 p.m.**

Bed. Muscles heavy. Mind loud, then quiet.

Emergency medicine gives you clarity — immediate feedback, sharp purpose. It also takes something every shift. Not all at once. Just enough to notice.

In the dark, Sam thinks:

*I can do this well. The question is how long doing it well costs less than it gives.*

The next shift is already on the calendar.

Chapter 14

# Day In The Life -- Orthopedics

**04:39 a.m.**

The alarm goes off early because orthopedics doesn't wait for anyone. Alex Morgan, PA-C is already half-awake when it sounds, body tuned to OR mornings. Today is a split day — **clinic in the morning, surgery in the afternoon** — the kind of schedule that looks balanced on paper and feels relentless in practice.

Tank, a ninety-pound German Shepherd with anxiety issues and opinions, is pacing the hallway like he's late for rounds. A fish tank glows softly in the living room — six neon tetras drifting, oblivious to surgical schedules.

"Relax," Alex mutters, swinging out of bed. "We're on time."

**04:48 a.m.**

Coffee goes on. Breakfast is high-protein by design: two hard-boiled eggs, oatmeal with peanut butter, eaten standing up. Ortho days burn calories whether you mean them to or not.

Alex works **Orthopedic Surgery**, five years in, mostly joints and sports injuries. The supervising physician, Dr. Reynolds, MD, expects competence, efficiency, and zero drama. Teaching happens, but not gently.

Scrubs for clinic now. OR scrubs later.

**05:27 a.m.**

Tank is fed. The fish get flakes. Alex checks the OR schedule on the phone: two total knees, one rotator cuff repair. No surprises. That's never true.

**05:49 a.m.**

Drive in. Dark roads. Construction cones. Alex runs through implant trays and positioning in their head like a checklist. Forgetting things in ortho isn't theoretical — it costs time, money, and trust.

**06:21 a.m.**

Clinic doors open. Charts already stacked.

Dr. Reynolds is down the hall, dictating at a speed Alex has never fully adjusted to. They exchange a nod. No small talk.

**06:34 a.m.**

First patient: post-op knee replacement. Alex removes the dressing, checks the incision (gl), range of motion (gl), swelling. It looks good. Not perfect. Good is enough.

"How's PT?" Alex asks.

The patient groans. "Hate it."

"Good," Alex says evenly. "That means it's working."

Education. Expectations. Documentation.

**07:19 a.m.**

New consult: ACL tear (gl). MRI reviewed. Alex explains anatomy with a model, walks through surgical vs conservative options. The patient asks about recovery time. Alex answers honestly. No sugarcoating. Ortho patients need clarity, not comfort.

**08:06 a.m.**

Dr. Reynolds steps into the room midway. He listens. Corrects one detail. Confirms the plan.

“You good with that?” he asks the patient.

“Yes.”

Dr. Reynolds looks at Alex. “Schedule it.”

Trust is quiet in ortho. It shows up as delegation.

**09:42 a.m.**

Fracture follow-up. X-rays (gl) pulled up. Healing slower than expected.

Alex flags Dr. Reynolds.

“Alignment’s off,” Alex says.

Dr. Reynolds squints. “Yeah. Might need revision.”

Alex feels the weight. This is where decisions ripple.

**10:31 a.m.**

Clinic wraps late. Alex inhales a protein bar and water while changing into OR scrubs. No lunch break. No illusion of one.

**11:07 a.m.**

OR. Bright. Cold. Controlled chaos.

Alex scrubs in with muscle memory. Dr. Reynolds arrives focused, already mentally inside the knee.

**11:26 a.m.**

Incision made. Alex assists — retracting, suctioning, positioning. Hours pass measured in millimeters and pressure.

Dr. Reynolds doesn't explain much. He doesn't need to. Alex anticipates the next instrument, the next move. When Alex hesitates once, Dr. Reynolds corrects sharply.

"Don't fight the joint."

Alex adjusts. Learns. Keeps going.

**01:48 p.m.**

Second case. Shoulder. Less blood. More precision. Alex holds tension for long stretches, forearms burning.

This is the physical toll people don't mention.

**03:32 p.m.**

Cases finish. Alex helps close, applies dressings, writes post-op orders. Dr. Reynolds leaves without ceremony.

"Good work," he says at the door. That's it. That's praise.

**04:11 p.m.**

Post-op rounds. Alex checks on patients waking from anesthesia. Pain control questions. Family explanations. The emotional work returns here.

**05:03 p.m.**

Paperwork. Consents. Notes. Implant documentation. Ortho paperwork is unforgiving.

**05:46 p.m.**

Locker room. Alex peels off OR scrubs, muscles aching in quiet protest.

**06:08 p.m.**

Drive home. Silence. Hands still feel like they're gripping instruments.

**06:31 p.m.**

Home. Tank explodes with joy, nearly knocking Alex over. The fish remain unimpressed.

Dinner is leftovers eaten on the couch, legs stretched out. Ice pack on one shoulder.

**08:47 p.m.**

Alex scrolls tomorrow's schedule. More clinic. No OR.

Relief and disappointment coexist.

In bed, Alex thinks:

*I like the clarity. I like the precision. I don't love how much of my body this job requires.*

The alarm is set again.

Chapter 15

# Day In The Life - - General Surgery

**03:58 a.m.**

The alarm goes off in the dark, not because it's humane, but because surgery doesn't care. Morgan Lee, PA-C opens their eyes and lies still for one full breath, orienting. General surgery days start before the rest of the hospital is honest about being awake.

Atlas, a lean, aging border collie with cloudy eyes and impeccable timing, rises from the rug and stretches like this is a shared mission. No cat. No fish. Just the dog and the early hour.

"Alright," Morgan says quietly. "Rounds."

**04:07 a.m.**

Coffee. Black. Breakfast is a protein shake and a banana — anything that won't fight back later. Morgan works **General Surgery**, seven years in, split between inpatient service, OR, and consults. The supervising physicians rotate, but the expectations don't: know the patients, know the plan, don't miss anything.

Scrubs on. Hair secured. Badge clipped. Morgan checks the census on their phone while drinking the last swallow of coffee.

Twenty-three patients. Three fresh post-ops. Two possible add-ons.

**04:41 a.m.**

Drive in. Roads empty. Morgan runs the list in their head — bowel resection in 412, cholecystectomy in 427, complicated appendectomy admitted overnight with rising white count (gl). Someone's going to turn.

**05:06 a.m.**

Hospital entrance. Badge swipe. Elevators smell like disinfectant and fatigue.

**05:14 a.m.**

Pre-rounds. Morgan moves room to room quietly, reviewing vitals, drains (gl), incisions (gl), pain control, urine output (gl). This is where PAs earn their keep — catching problems before they announce themselves.

In 412, Morgan pauses. The patient looks off. Slight tachycardia (gl). Drain output higher than expected.

Morgan makes a note and flags it mentally.

**06:02 a.m.**

Team rounds. Two attendings today. One resident. Morgan stands at the computer, ready.

Dr. Feldman, MD runs the list fast.

"412?"

"Concern for leak," Morgan says. "Drain output's up. Vitals trending."

Dr. Feldman nods. "CT this morning. NPO. Broad-spectrum antibiotics."

"Already ordered," Morgan replies.

That's the dynamic. Anticipation matters.

**06:41 a.m.**

OR time. Morgan changes into OR scrubs, scrubs in alongside Dr. Chen, MD for the first case — laparoscopic cholecystectomy (gl).

The case is smooth until it isn't. Anatomy distorted. Adhesions (gl). Morgan retracts, suctions, adjusts. Dr. Chen works silently, focused.

When Morgan anticipates the next step correctly, Dr. Chen nods once. That's approval.

**08:19 a.m.**

Case done. Closure. Dressings. Orders. Morgan moves fast — the floor doesn't wait.

**08:47 a.m.**

Consult pager goes off. Abdominal pain in the ED. Morgan heads down, reviews imaging, examines the patient. Guarding (gl). Rebound (gl). Appendicitis (gl), but complicated.

Morgan calls Dr. Feldman.

"Likely surgical. I'd book."

"Agree. Get consent. We'll add on."

Another ripple added to the day.

**10:06 a.m.**

Post-op checks. Pain management adjustments. Family questions. Morgan explains what surgeons don't always have time to — timelines, expectations, what's normal and what's not.

**11:22 a.m.**

The patient in 412 spikes a fever.

Morgan doesn't wait. Labs ordered. Imaging expedited. Dr. Feldman notified.

This is where experience shows — not in heroics, but in speed.

**12:08 p.m.**

Lunch is theoretical. Morgan drinks half a protein shake while charting standing up.

**12:31 p.m.**

Back to the OR. Add-on appendectomy. This one bleeds more than expected. Morgan's forearms burn holding tension. The room is quiet except for suction.

**02:14 p.m.**

Case ends. Morgan helps close, strips gloves, feels the fatigue hit late.

**02:47 p.m.**

Back upstairs. The CT confirms a leak in 412.

Morgan briefs Dr. Feldman.

"We need to take them back."

Dr. Feldman sighs. "Book it."

The day reshapes itself again.

**03:36 p.m.**

Consent discussion. Hard one. Risks. Uncertainty. Family frightened.

Morgan answers questions honestly, calmly. This isn't the OR. This is the human part.

**05:02 p.m.**

Back in the OR. Second operation on the same patient. Stakes higher now. Morgan assists, focused, steady.

**06:48 p.m.**

Case finishes. The patient goes to ICU.

Morgan documents meticulously. Every detail matters later.

**07:31 p.m.**

Sign-out. Clean. Thorough. Morgan hands the list to the night PA, flags concerns.

**07:52 p.m.**

Locker room. Scrubs off. Hands washed until the smell of betadine finally fades.

**08:13 p.m.**

Drive home. The sky is dark again. The loop is complete.

**08:36 p.m.**

Home. Atlas greets Morgan with slow, happy circles. Dinner is leftovers eaten standing up while leaning on the counter.

**09:41 p.m.**

Morgan sits on the floor with Atlas, back against the couch, finally still.

General surgery offers intensity, clarity, and purpose — and it takes stamina, flexibility, and a tolerance for unfinished days.

In the quiet, Morgan thinks:

*I like being needed. I don't like how often that need erases the rest of the day.*

The alarm is already set.

Chapter 16

# Day In The Life - - Specialty Clinic (Pulmonology)

**05:32 a.m.**

The house is quiet in the way it only is before people start needing oxygen.

Evan Brooks, PA-C sits up slowly, testing his own breath before he even thinks about patients'. Old habit. Not anxiety — calibration.

A yellow lab named Moose thumps his tail once against the wall, still half asleep. No rush yet.

Evan is a **career outpatient pulmonology Physician Assistant**, twelve years into practice. COPD (gl), asthma (gl), interstitial lung disease (gl) — chronic, progressive, often invisible to anyone who hasn't watched someone struggle for air.

He didn't choose this specialty for excitement. He chose it because breath is fundamental, and people underestimate how terrifying it is to lose.

**05:41 a.m.**

Coffee. Breakfast is eggs and toast, eaten sitting down. Evan refuses to start days rushed — pulmonary patients feel time pressure immediately.

Scrubs are light blue. Badge clipped. Pulse oximeter (gl) already in his pocket out of reflex.

**06:19 a.m.**

Drive in. Evan notices his own breathing syncing with the car's movement. Slow. Controlled. He'll need that today.

**06:52 a.m.**

Clinic opens. The waiting room is full of people who look fine — until they move.

Dr. Kline, MD — supervising pulmonologist — is reviewing CT scans (gl). They've worked together for nearly a decade. Pulmonology is a thinking specialty; their collaboration reflects that.

"I've got a new ILD consult at ten," Evan says.

Dr. Kline nods. "I'll want eyes on that."

**07:14 a.m.**

First patient. Severe asthma follow-up. Controller medication adherence poor. Rescue inhaler used daily.

Evan doesn't scold. He demonstrates inhaler technique (gl) again. Half the problem lives there.

The patient breathes easier by the end — partly physiologic, partly psychological.

**08:32 a.m.**

COPD visit. Oxygen-dependent (gl). The patient hates the tubing, the stigma, the limits.

Evan adjusts flow rates, reviews exertional dyspnea (gl), and talks about pacing. Pulmonology isn't about cure. It's about making life tolerable.

**09:48 a.m.**

Pulmonary function testing (gl) review. Numbers trending down. Evan explains what they mean — and what they don't.

"We're watching change," he says. "Not judging you."

That sentence matters.

**10:57 a.m.**

New consult. Interstitial lung disease suspected. CT images up on the screen.

Evan feels the weight immediately. These conversations are slow burns.

He steps out, pulls Dr. Kline in.

"I think we're early — but not early enough."

Dr. Kline nods. "Let's talk biopsy timing."

They return together. That matters to patients.

**12:14 p.m.**

Lunch exists, technically. Evan eats while documenting, careful with phrasing. Pulmonary notes age poorly if you're sloppy.

**01:09 p.m.**

Sleep apnea (gl) follow-up. CPAP compliance poor. The patient is frustrated.

Evan reframes. Different mask. Different settings. Different expectations.

Breathing at night is as emotional as it is mechanical.

**02:41 p.m.**

Shortness of breath visit. The patient insists it's "just getting older."

Evan listens, examines, orders imaging. Experience tells him this is cardiac overlap (gl), not pulmonary.

He coordinates care instead of defending turf.

**03:56 p.m.**

Last patient. Long-term smoker. Lung nodules (gl) under surveillance.

Evan explains watchful waiting without minimizing fear. That balance takes years to learn.

**04:38 p.m.**

Charts closed. Imaging requests sent. Follow-ups scheduled months out — pulmonary time moves differently.

Dr. Kline passes by. "Thanks for handling the ILD consult."

Evan nods. He'll feel that one later.

**05:07 p.m.**

Drive home. Evan notices he's breathing shallow again. He fixes it consciously.

**05:32 p.m.**

Moose greets him like he's been gone forever. Dinner is quiet. Evan doesn't talk much.

Later, lying in bed, he thinks:

*People think lungs fail loudly. Mostly, they fade.*

He turns onto his side, one hand resting on his own chest — feeling the rise, the fall — grateful, and a little haunted.

Chapter 17

# Day In The Life -- Surgical First Assist (OR Day)

**04:11 a.m.**

The alarm is sharp because the day will be, too. Riley Chen, PA-C doesn't open their eyes right away. OR days require a brief mental inventory before the body joins the conversation. First assist today. Three cases scheduled. Two more likely.

Koda, a young black lab with boundless optimism, springs off the bed as if the alarm were for him. He skids into the doorframe, recovers, and looks back proudly. A fish tank glows blue in the corner of the living room, steady and indifferent.

"Easy," Riley says, already smiling despite the hour.

**04:20 a.m.**

Coffee. Strong. Breakfast is deliberate and boring: oatmeal with peanut butter and a hard-boiled egg. First assist days are physical; hunger shows up as hand tremor if you're careless.

Riley works **as a Surgical First Assist**, seven years in practice, credentialed across multiple services. Today's list:

general surgery and vascular. Same building. Different expectations.

Scrubs laid out. Compression socks on. Hair secured tight. Hands already feel like tools.

**04:54 a.m.**

Drive in. Dark roads, construction barrels, the low hum of anticipation. No music. Riley visualizes cases instead — incision points, positioning, where the surgeon will want the retractor held without asking.

**05:22 a.m.**

OR locker room. Change into hospital scrubs. Badge clipped. Riley checks the board: rooms already turning over.

Dr. Hargreeve, MD — lead surgeon for the morning — is reviewing images at the workstation, jaw set.

“Morning,” Riley says.

Dr. Hargreeve nods. “You’re with me all day.”

That’s confirmation and expectation in one sentence.

**05:41 a.m.**

First case setup. Positioning matters. Padding pressure points. Confirming laterality. Riley double-checks everything. First assist lives in the margin between smooth and catastrophic.

**06:02 a.m.**

Scrub in. The water is cold. Riley runs through the ritual precisely — nails, fingers, forearms — then steps into the room as the sterile field comes together.

**06:14 a.m.**

Incision.

Riley retracts, suctions, exposes. The job is to make the surgeon's work possible without being noticed. When Riley adjusts without being asked, Dr. Hargreeve says nothing. That's success.

Minutes stretch. Muscles engage and stay engaged. This is not finesse; it's endurance.

**07:43 a.m.**

Closure. Riley assists with suturing (gl), layers clean and even. The case ends quietly.

No applause. No discussion. Just efficiency.

**08:01 a.m.**

Room turnover. Riley drinks water, eats half a protein bar, re-ties hair. The second case is already rolling.

**08:27 a.m.**

Vascular case. Different energy. Higher stakes.

Riley holds steady pressure on a vessel for long minutes while Dr. Hargreeve works millimeters away. Forearms burn. Shoulders protest. Riley adjusts stance, breath, grip — anything but the field.

At one point, Riley anticipates a clamp and has it ready. Dr. Hargreeve glances once.

"Good," he says.

That single word lands heavier than praise.

**10:46 a.m.**

Case complete. Riley helps dress the incision, steps back as anesthesia lightens sedation. Another patient handed off.

**11:02 a.m.**

Third case delayed. Equipment issue. Riley waits in the substerile room, stretching fingers, shaking out shoulders. First assist work is invisible until your body reminds you it isn't.

**11:34 a.m.**

Add-on case confirmed. Of course it is.

**12:07 p.m.**

Back in the room. Scrub in again. This case runs long.

Riley stands almost motionless for stretches that erase the sense of time. Sweat pools under the cap. Hands remain steady. That's the job.

**02:51 p.m.**

Final closure. Riley helps clean, de-drape, document.

Dr. Hargreeve peels off gloves. "Thanks for today."

It's not warmth. It's acknowledgment.

**03:18 p.m.**

OR day is technically done. Riley signs out, changes, stretches slowly in the locker room. Legs ache. Back tight. This work taxes the body first and asks questions later.

**03:47 p.m.**

Drive home early by hospital standards, late by circadian ones. Sun still high. The rest of the world is mid-day; Riley feels like it should be evening.

**04:06 p.m.**

Home. Koda greets Riley like a miracle has occurred. The fish remain unimpressed.

Dinner is early, simple, eaten sitting down for once. Riley's hands finally unclench.

**06:22 p.m.**

Ice pack on one shoulder. Stretching on the floor. The body recovers in pieces.

First assist days are satisfying in a specific way — clean lines, defined roles, no ambiguity about who decides. They're also transactional with the body.

As the light fades, Riley thinks:

*I like knowing exactly where I fit. I don't love how much standing in that place costs.*

Tomorrow is clinic.

The alarm is already set.

Chapter 18

# Day In The Life -- Inpatient Hospital Medicine

**05:23 a.m.**

The alarm goes off in that half-hour where the body doesn't know whether it's night or morning. Taylor Brooks, PA-C rolls onto their side, already aware of the weight waiting at the hospital.

This is a **hospital medicine day shift** — census heavy, discharges stacked, consults trickling in all day whether the board looks full or not.

Milo, a sleepy beagle with selective hearing, lifts his head long enough to confirm movement, then drops it back onto the blanket. A cat named Pepper weaves between Taylor's legs as they stand, already demanding breakfast before logic has fully loaded.

**05:31 a.m.**

Coffee first. Breakfast is oatmeal with berries, eaten slowly on purpose. Hospital medicine punishes rushing later.

Taylor has been a **Hospital Medicine PA** for four years. The work is less dramatic than the ED, less procedural than surgery, and more cognitively relentless than either. The supervising physicians rotate weekly. The expectations don't.

Scrubs on. Badge clipped. Laptop bag packed. Taylor checks the patient list on the phone: eighteen patients assigned. Three new admissions overnight.

**06:02 a.m.**

Drive in. Early commuters. School buses warming up. Taylor reviews overnight notes mentally — one pneumonia (gl), one heart failure (gl) exacerbation, one patient with unclear abdominal pain who's probably going to need imaging.

**06:34 a.m.**

Hospital entrance. Badge swipe. Elevators already full of tired faces.

**06:42 a.m.**

Pre-rounding starts immediately. Taylor moves room to room, scanning vitals, labs, overnight events. This is detective work, not showmanship.

In room 714, oxygen requirements crept up overnight. Taylor makes a note.

In 721, creatinine (gl) jumped. That will need adjusting before rounds.

**07:21 a.m.**

Team huddle. Dr. Lawson, MD — attending for the week — reviews the list.

Taylor speaks when it matters.

"714's oxygen increased. I'm concerned we're not turning the corner."

Dr. Lawson nods. "Let's escalate imaging."

This is shared cognition. It's quiet and essential.

**07:58 a.m.**

Formal rounds. Taylor walks with the team, presenting patients succinctly, answering questions, adjusting plans in real time. When the plan is clear, Taylor executes it. Orders fly. Consults placed. Discharge planning initiated before anyone asks.

**09:34 a.m.**

Family meeting. A patient's daughter is overwhelmed, angry, scared. Taylor explains heart failure in plain language, sets expectations gently, answers questions the attending doesn't have time to linger on.

This is where hospital medicine lives — in translation.

**10:47 a.m.**

Discharge number one. Med reconciliation (gl) takes longer than expected. Insurance delays threaten to stall it. Taylor calls case management, pharmacy, the patient's outpatient provider. The system resists. Taylor persists.

**11:58 a.m.**

Admission from the ED. Sepsis (gl) rule-out. Taylor reviews imaging, labs, history, then calls Dr. Lawson.

"I think this is early sepsis. Fluids are in. Antibiotics started. We need close monitoring."

"Agreed," Dr. Lawson says. "Put them on telemetry."

Taylor places the orders.

**12:26 p.m.**

Lunch exists on paper. In practice, it's yogurt eaten while charting.

**01:19 p.m.**

Consult from cardiology. Adjust beta blockers (gl). Update the plan. Document thoroughly. Hospital medicine is documentation-forward — every word protects continuity.

**02:08 p.m.**

Another discharge stalls. Home oxygen not approved yet. The patient is frustrated. Taylor explains the delay, absorbs the anger without taking it personally.

**03:14 p.m.**

Rapid response overhead. Not Taylor's patient — but Taylor steps in anyway, helps gather supplies, supports the team. Inpatient work is communal whether you want it to be or not.

**04:03 p.m.**

Back to the list. Notes incomplete. Labs still rolling in. Taylor double-checks everything now — fatigue breeds errors.

**05:21 p.m.**

Evening handoff prep. Taylor updates each patient succinctly, flags concerns, anticipates overnight issues.

Dr. Lawson stops by. “Good work today.”

It matters more than it should.

**05:54 p.m.**

Sign-out. Clean. No surprises. That’s the goal.

**06:11 p.m.**

Drive home. The brain is tired in a different way — not adrenaline-drained, but decision-heavy.

**06:34 p.m.**

Home. Milo greets Taylor with exaggerated enthusiasm. Pepper demands dinner immediately, as if this delay were criminal.

Dinner is simple. Conversation minimal. The day doesn’t need retelling.

**09:02 p.m.**

Laptop closed. Tomorrow’s list already posted. Taylor doesn’t look.

Hospital medicine offers rhythm, continuity, and intellectual satisfaction — and it demands patience with a system that moves slower than illness.

In the quiet, Taylor thinks:

*I like being the steady one. I don’t love how invisible that steadiness can be.*

The alarm is set.

Chapter 19

# Day In The Life - - ICU (Consult / Service Support)

**04:28 a.m.**

The alarm cuts through sleep like a blade. ICU days don't ease you in; they assume readiness. Chris Alvarez, PA-C opens their eyes and takes one steadying breath before moving. The unit doesn't care how rested you are. It cares how sharp you are.

Nico, a compact blue heeler with endless energy and terrible timing, skids across the floor the second Chris sits up. A cat named Solstice remains curled into a tight, indifferent comma at the foot of the bed.

"Not today," Chris murmurs, stepping over Nico and heading for the kitchen.

**04:36 a.m.**

Coffee goes on. Breakfast is deliberate: eggs, toast, and a protein shake. ICU work punishes low blood sugar and sloppy thinking equally.

Chris works **ICU consult/service support**, six years in practice, split between critical care consults and co-management. The supervising intensivists rotate; the standard doesn't. The expectation is clear: catch problems early, escalate without ego, and never assume stability is permanent.

Scrubs on. Badge clipped. Laptop bag zipped. Chris checks overnight alerts — vent alarms (gl), vasopressor (gl) titrations, labs flagged critical.

**05:11 a.m.**

Drive in. Dark roads. No music. The brain needs room.

Chris mentally reviews the unit census: ARDS (gl) in bed 9, septic shock (gl) in 12, post-op GI bleed in 4. None of them slept. Neither will the team.

**05:43 a.m.**

Badge swipe. The ICU hums constantly — ventilators, pumps, monitors speaking in numbers and tones that become a second language.

The night PA gives sign-out fast and clean. "Bed 12's MAP (gl) dipped twice. Pressors adjusted. Bed 9 desatted at 4 a.m. Improved with suctioning."

Chris nods. That's enough to start.

**06:02 a.m.**

Pre-rounds. Chris moves bed to bed, eyes scanning monitors before faces. In the ICU, the numbers tell the story before the patient can.

Bed 12 looks worse. Skin mottled. Lactate (gl) still climbing.

Chris adjusts the plan in their head before touching the chart.

**06:41 a.m.**

Rounds begin. Dr. Simmons, MD — attending intensivist — leads. Chris presents succinctly, anticipating questions.

"I'm concerned about escalating vasopressor needs and worsening acidosis (gl). We may need additional support."

Dr. Simmons nods. "Agreed. Let's add vasopressin and get another ABG (gl)."

Orders placed immediately. Time matters here.

**07:18 a.m.**

A ventilator alarm sounds from across the unit. Chris moves before it finishes beeping. Secretions. Hypoxia (gl). Suctioning improves sats.

The patient doesn't wake. The family watches, terrified.

Chris explains what just happened in plain language. This is part of the job no monitor tracks.

**08:02 a.m.**

Consult from surgery. Post-op patient borderline unstable. Chris reviews imaging, labs, trends.

Chris calls Dr. Simmons.

"This isn't just pain. I think we're missing early sepsis."

"Bring them to the unit," Dr. Simmons says. "I'll meet you there."

The escalation is clean. No resistance.

**09:41 a.m.**

Family meeting. Ventilator. Prognosis uncertain. Chris sits with them, answers questions carefully, avoids false reassurance. ICU honesty is its own discipline.

**10:53 a.m.**

Lines adjusted. Drips titrated. Chris coordinates with nursing, respiratory therapy, pharmacy. ICU care is orchestration.

**12:06 p.m.**

Lunch exists in theory. Chris drinks a protein shake while charting, eyes never fully leaving the monitors.

**12:49 p.m.**

Bed 12 crashes.

Blood pressure drops. Heart rate spikes. Chris calls out orders while moving — fluids, pressors, labs. Dr. Simmons arrives immediately. The room fills.

Chris manages access, communicates changes, documents in real time. This is where training shows.

**01:27 p.m.**

The patient stabilizes — for now.

Chris steps out of the room, hands trembling slightly. They notice. They don't comment.

**02:18 p.m.**

Back to consults. Adjust sedation (gl). Reassess vent settings. ICU work never stops. It just shifts intensity.

**03:44 p.m.**

Another family meeting. Different patient. Same fear.

Chris answers the question that never feels fair: "Are they going to make it?"

Chris answers honestly: "I don't know yet. We're doing everything we can."

**04:52 p.m.**

Afternoon labs reviewed. Plans adjusted. Chris prepares sign-out meticulously. In the ICU, sloppy handoffs cost lives.

**06:01 p.m.**

Evening handoff. Clean. Detailed. No assumptions.

Dr. Simmons stops Chris before leaving. "Good catches today."

It lands heavier than praise elsewhere.

**06:24 p.m.**

Drive home. The adrenaline drains late. The day lingers in fragments — alarms, numbers, faces.

**06:47 p.m.**

Home. Nico greets Chris like survival has been confirmed. Solstice flicks her tail.

Dinner is quiet. The TV stays off. The nervous system needs dark and still.

**09:11 p.m.**

Bed. The hum of monitors echoes faintly in memory, then fades.

ICU work offers intensity, precision, and immediate impact — and it asks you to carry outcomes that don't always resolve cleanly.

In the dark, Chris thinks:

*I can manage the chaos. The question is how many days like this my body agrees to.*

The alarm is already set.

Chapter 20

# Day In The Life -- Pediatrics

**05:18 a.m.**

The alarm goes off softly because the day will be loud enough on its own. Elena Ruiz, PA-C opens her eyes and smiles before she sits up — not because she's rested, but because pediatrics is the one place in medicine where smiling before coffee sometimes makes sense.

Piper, a small tri-color corgi with permanent side-eye, hops off the bed and spins in a tight circle. A parakeet named Blue starts chirping from the living room like the alarm was his idea.

"Too early," Elena says, but she's already up.

Elena is a **full-time Pediatrics Physician Assistant**, eight years into practice, entirely outpatient. She didn't "end up" here. She chose it, deliberately, after deciding early in her career that she wanted continuity, long arcs, and relationships that spanned years instead of encounters.

**05:26 a.m.**

Coffee. Breakfast is yogurt with granola and berries, eaten sitting down — a non-negotiable rule Elena learned the hard way. Pediatrics requires patience, and patience runs on glucose.

Scrubs are cheerful but not childish. Badge clipped. Stethoscope around her neck — pediatric-sized diaphragm. Elena checks the schedule on her phone.

Twenty-two kids today. Four well-child visits. Three behavioral follow-ups. Two "same-day sick" slots that will absolutely be used.

**05:58 a.m.**

Drive in. Morning radio low. Elena mentally reviews names, not diagnoses. That's how pediatrics works. These aren't "cases." They're kids she's known since infancy.

**06:29 a.m.**

Clinic doors open. The waiting room already smells faintly of disinfectant and apple juice.

Dr. Howard, MD — supervising pediatrician — is in his office reviewing charts. He's worked with Elena for six years. Their dynamic is steady, collaborative, and boring in the best possible way.

"Morning," he says.

"Morning," Elena replies. "I've got the Martinez twins first."

He winces. "Godspeed."

They both smile.

**07:02 a.m.**

First room. Two toddlers. One parent. Chaos contained only by goldfish crackers.

Elena crouches to eye level immediately. “Hi, I’m Elena. Can I listen to your heart?”

One child says no. The other tries to eat the stethoscope.

This is normal.

Vitals, growth curves, vaccines (gl). Elena explains what’s coming before it happens — to the parents *and* the kids. That’s the trick. No surprises.

**08:11 a.m.**

Well-child visit. Eight years old. Elena notices the kid has dropped percentile on the growth chart (gl). Subtle. Easy to miss.

She asks questions gently. Appetite. Sleep. Stress. School.

The answer comes sideways. Bullying. Stomachaches that aren’t GI.

Elena documents carefully and flags it for follow-up. Pediatrics is pattern recognition over time.

**09:26 a.m.**

Sick visit. Fever. Sore throat. Rapid strep (gl) positive.

Elena explains antibiotics to the parent and responsibility to the child. “You take this every day. Even when you feel better.”

The child nods solemnly.

**10:14 a.m.**

Behavioral follow-up. ADHD (gl). Medication titration. School reports reviewed.

Elena loops Dr. Howard in briefly.

"Thinking small increase," she says.

"Agree," he replies. "Monitor sleep."

That's it. No power struggle. Just alignment.

**11:38 a.m.**

Lunch exists today. Elena eats half a sandwich while charting, then actually finishes the other half. Victory.

**12:22 p.m.**

Same-day sick slot. Infant. Parent terrified. Breathing sounds wrong.

Elena listens carefully. RSV (gl) season. Mild retractions (gl), but sats okay.

She explains warning signs slowly, clearly. Writes them down. Pediatrics is reassurance *with guardrails*.

**01:41 p.m.**

Teen visit. Door closed. Parent outside.

Mental health screening (gl). Elena asks the questions directly. No euphemisms. No judgment.

The answers are honest. Elena thanks them for trusting her.

This is why she stays in pediatrics.

**03:08 p.m.**

Last patient. A kid Elena has seen since birth. Height chart looks good. Confidence higher than last year. Elena notices.

“You seem taller,” she says.

The kid beams.

**04:27 p.m.**

Notes done. Inbox cleared. Vaccine inventory checked for tomorrow.

Dr. Howard stops by. “Nice catch on the growth chart earlier.”

Elena nods. That matters here.

**04:56 p.m.**

Drive home. Daylight still out. The emotional residue is lighter today — not absent, but lighter.

**05:18 p.m.**

Home. Piper greets Elena like she’s been gone for months. Blue chirps approval.

Dinner is real. Conversation is light. Elena doesn’t replay charts in her head the way she used to earlier in her career.

**08:49 p.m.**

Elena sets out scrubs for tomorrow. Same clinic. Same kids. New problems.

In bed, she thinks:

*I don't save lives every day. I shape them. That's enough for me.*

I don't take charts to bed — but some stories try to come anyway.

The alarm is set.

Chapter 21

# Day In The Life -- Psychiatry / Behavioral Health

**06:04 a.m.**

The alarm goes off gently because the work won't be. Maya Thompson, PA-C lies still for a moment, letting her nervous system come online slowly. Psychiatry days demand presence, not adrenaline.

Otis, a senior mixed-breed rescue with cloudy eyes and impeccable manners, lifts his head and waits. He has learned that rushing doesn't help mornings like this.

Maya works **full-time in outpatient psychiatry**, nine years into practice. She chose this lane after learning early that she was good at procedures — and better at sitting with people when there was nothing to *do* except listen.

**06:12 a.m.**

Coffee. Breakfast is toast with almond butter and a hard-boiled egg, eaten at the table. Maya never eats standing up on workdays. Small rituals keep the day from leaking into her.

Scrubs aren't required here. She dresses professionally but softly — fabrics that don't distract, colors that don't announce authority. Badge clipped. Notebook in bag.

**06:47 a.m.**

Drive in. Quiet playlist, low volume. Maya reviews the schedule mentally: medication management, therapy-adjacent visits, one new patient intake that will likely run long.

Psychiatry punishes rigidity. She leaves space.

**07:21 a.m.**

Clinic opens. The waiting room is subdued — no coughs, no children, just people staring at their phones like shields.

Dr. Kaplan, MD — supervising psychiatrist — is already in his office, door open. He and Maya have worked together for seven years. Their relationship is steady, consultative, built on trust.

"Morning," he says.

"Morning," Maya replies. "I may grab you for the new intake later."

"Of course," he says. No questions.

**07:42 a.m.**

First patient. Follow-up for major depressive disorder (gl). Medication review. Sleep still fragmented. Appetite poor.

Maya doesn't rush. She asks open questions and waits through the silence that makes other clinicians uncomfortable. The patient eventually fills it.

They adjust the plan slightly. No big swings. Psychiatry is incremental by design.

**08:51 a.m.**

Anxiety disorder (gl). Panic symptoms improving, but work stress escalating. Maya discusses coping strategies, validates the difficulty, and reinforces boundaries.

She documents carefully. Words matter here more than anywhere else.

**10:03 a.m.**

New patient intake. The room feels heavier the moment Maya sits down. Trauma history. Multiple diagnoses. Med list long and messy.

Maya listens for forty minutes before offering anything. When she does speak, it's precise.

"I want to understand what's helped before — and what hasn't," she says.

The patient exhales like they've been holding their breath for years.

**11:26 a.m.**

Maya steps out and grabs Dr. Kaplan.

"This is complex," she says quietly. "I'm thinking we simplify before we add."

Dr. Kaplan reviews the chart, nods. "Agreed. You want to co-manage initially?"

"Yes."

"Done."

That's supervision in psychiatry — collaboration, not oversight theater.

**12:18 p.m.**

Lunch. Actually eaten. Salad and soup at her desk, door closed. Maya reads something non-medical on purpose.

**01:07 p.m.**

Afternoon follow-ups. Bipolar disorder (gl). Mood stable but sleep drifting. Medication adherence discussed honestly. No shaming.

Maya checks labs, reviews side effects, documents risk assessment (gl). This is quiet work with high stakes.

**02:29 p.m.**

A patient arrives visibly distressed. Passive suicidal ideation (gl) disclosed.

Maya's posture shifts immediately — not alarmed, just anchored. She asks the questions directly, without euphemism.

"Are you thinking about harming yourself?"

The answer is complicated. Maya stays with it. Safety planning begins. Dr. Kaplan joins the room midway. Together, they decide on next steps.

This is why psychiatry days are draining even when nothing "happens."

**04:03 p.m.**

Notes. Care coordination. Follow-up calls. Psychiatry extends beyond the room.

**04:47 p.m.**

Last chart closed. Maya pauses before shutting down the computer. She checks herself — tension in shoulders, jaw tight. She releases both intentionally.

Dr. Kaplan passes by. “Good work today.”

Maya nods. It means he saw the hard parts.

**05:11 p.m.**

Drive home. Music off. Windows cracked. Maya doesn’t replay conversations anymore — that took training.

**05:34 p.m.**

Home. Otis greets her slowly, tail wagging like punctuation. Dinner is simple. Conversation light.

**08:58 p.m.**

Maya writes tomorrow’s first patient name on a sticky note, then closes the notebook. She doesn’t bring charts to bed.

In the quiet, she thinks:

*I don’t fix people. I walk with them while they learn how to carry themselves.*

The alarm is set.

Chapter 22

# Day in the Life — Women's Health / OB-GYN

**05:06 a.m.**

The alarm goes off once and that's enough. Claire Donovan, PA-C opens her eyes already tracking where she is in the week. Clinic-heavy day. Procedures scheduled. No deliveries — but OB-GYN days have a way of changing their minds.

Hazel, a lean gray whippet with permanent anxiety and Olympic-level speed, jumps off the bed and paces the hallway like something urgent has been announced. A calico cat named Marigold remains curled in the chair, tail flicking once in mild disapproval.

"Give me a minute," Claire says, voice soft but firm. Boundaries start early in this specialty.

Claire is a **Women's Health / OB-GYN Physician Assistant**, ten years into practice, primarily outpatient with procedural days mixed in. She chose this field for the blend of continuity, autonomy, and advocacy — and learned quickly that it requires emotional stamina more than technical bravado.

**05:14 a.m.**

Coffee. Breakfast is deliberate: toast, peanut butter, and a hard-boiled egg eaten sitting down. OB-GYN is one of the few specialties where you will be asked about your tone as much as your plan.

Scrubs are clean and neutral. Badge clipped. Ultrasound reports reviewed on the phone before leaving. Two colposcopies (gl) today. One IUD insertion (gl). One difficult follow-up she's already thinking about.

**05:51 a.m.**

Drive in. Dawn just breaking. Claire keeps the radio off. She uses the drive to rehearse conversations — not procedures. That's the work that lingers.

**06:28 a.m.**

Clinic doors open. The waiting room is already filling — different ages, different reasons, same vulnerability.

Dr. Feldman, MD — supervising OB-GYN — is reviewing surgical schedules in her office. She and Claire have worked together for eight years. Their relationship is efficient, mutual, and deeply protective of patients.

"Morning," Dr. Feldman says.

"Morning. I'll grab you after the colpo on room three," Claire replies.

"Of course."

**07:01 a.m.**

First patient. Annual exam. Claire moves deliberately, narrating each step before it happens. Consent here is active, not implied.

Vitals. History. Exam. Claire notices tension immediately and adjusts her pace. OB-GYN teaches you to read micro-signals.

**08:12 a.m.**

Colposcopy. The patient is anxious, voice tight.

Claire explains again — slowly. Shows the instruments. Asks permission before each step. The procedure itself is routine. The emotional labor is not.

When it's done, the patient exhales like they've been underwater.

"You did great," Claire says, and means it.

**09:26 a.m.**

Contraception counseling. Long discussion. The patient is conflicted, worried about side effects, history complicated.

Claire doesn't steer. She clarifies. Options. Risks. Autonomy. This is where women's health either builds trust or loses it permanently.

**10:41 a.m.**

Follow-up for abnormal Pap smear (gl). Results reviewed. Next steps explained carefully. The patient's eyes fill before the word "cancer" is even said — and Claire makes sure it isn't.

Claire steps out briefly and updates Dr. Feldman.

"Low-grade. I'm thinking surveillance."

"Agree," Dr. Feldman says. "I'll cosign."

**11:58 a.m.**

Lunch is half a salad eaten while reviewing labs. Iron deficiency (gl). Thyroid levels (gl). Patterns emerging.

**12:37 p.m.**

IUD insertion. The patient is bracing for pain.

Claire prepares meticulously. Talks through breathing. Goes slowly. Stops when asked. When it's over, the patient laughs in relief.

"That wasn't as bad as I thought."

Claire smiles. "It never is when you're heard."

**01:49 p.m.**

Hard visit. Pregnancy loss. Not recent, but not healed.

Claire closes the door and gives the time this appointment actually needs, not what the schedule allows. She listens more than she speaks.

Some days, this is the whole job.

**03:18 p.m.**

Last patient. Teen visit. Mother in the room, eyes sharp. Claire navigates confidentiality carefully, explaining limits clearly.

Trust built now matters later.

**04:22 p.m.**

Charts closed. Procedure notes finalized. Follow-up plans scheduled.

Dr. Feldman stops by. “Thanks for handling that loss visit today.”

Claire nods. That recognition counts.

**04:51 p.m.**

Drive home. Emotional residue heavier than physical fatigue. Claire lets it ride instead of pushing it away.

**05:14 p.m.**

Home. Hazel explodes with joy. Marigold pretends nothing happened.

Dinner is quiet. Claire doesn’t talk much tonight.

**09:03 p.m.**

Scrubs laid out for tomorrow. A different mix of visits. Similar emotional demands.

In bed, Claire thinks:

*This work asks you to hold people at their most exposed. The cost is real — and so is the meaning.*

The alarm is set.

Chapter 23

# Day In The Life - - Specialty Clinic (Cardiology)

Chapter 24

# Day In The Life - - Specialty Clinic (Cardiology)

**05:02 a.m.**

The alarm goes off once, sharp and final. Cardiology days reward preparation and punish sloppiness. Marcus Hill, PA-C opens his eyes already thinking in numbers — heart rates, pressures, ejection fractions (gl).

Nova, a sleek black Doberman with guard-dog instincts and impeccable timing, lifts her head from the foot of the bed. No cat. No fish. Just the dog and the quiet expectation that Marcus will be useful today.

Marcus works **full-time in outpatient cardiology**, eleven years into practice. He didn't wander here. He built toward it — drawn by complexity, longitudinal care, and the uncomfortable truth that cardiac disease never stays theoretical.

**05:11 a.m.**

Coffee. Breakfast is oatmeal with berries and almonds, eaten slowly at the kitchen table while Marcus reviews overnight messages. Two hospital discharges. One patient with worsening dyspnea (gl). One abnormal Holter monitor (gl) flagged overnight.

Scrubs are neutral. Badge clipped. Stethoscope goes into the bag — cardiology still uses it daily, even when imaging dominates.

**05:47 a.m.**

Drive in. Dawn barely breaking. Marcus listens to nothing. He uses the drive to run through guideline thresholds and medication ladders in his head.

**06:21 a.m.**

Clinic opens. The waiting room is quiet in that particular way cardiology clinics are — people sitting still, aware that their problem is not abstract.

Dr. Singh, MD — supervising cardiologist — is already reviewing echo results. He and Marcus have worked together for nearly a decade. Their communication is efficient and exacting.

“Morning,” Dr. Singh says.

“Morning. I want to run a Holter with you before rooming,” Marcus replies.

They review it together. Runs of nonsustained ventricular tachycardia (gl). Not benign. Not emergent. Yet.

“Let’s bring him in sooner,” Dr. Singh says.

“Already scheduled,” Marcus replies.

That's the rhythm.

**07:04 a.m.**

First patient. Heart failure (gl) follow-up. Weight up three pounds. Ankles swollen. The patient insists they're "fine."

Marcus doesn't argue. He asks about sodium, fluid intake, missed doses. The answers tell the story.

Medication adjustment. Lab orders. Education delivered plainly, without fear tactics. Cardiology lives in the space between urgency and sustainability.

**08:19 a.m.**

Chest pain follow-up. Prior ED visit ruled out MI (gl), but symptoms persist.

Marcus reviews imaging, stress test (gl) results, labs. The picture is nuanced.

He steps into Dr. Singh's office.

"I don't think we're done here."

Dr. Singh nods. "CTA (gl). Let's look for something structural."

Plan confirmed. Marcus returns to the room and explains the why, not just the what.

**09:41 a.m.**

Atrial fibrillation (gl). Anticoagulation discussion. The patient is anxious about bleeding risk.

Marcus walks through risk stratification slowly, methodically. Numbers. Probabilities. Tradeoffs.

This is where trust either solidifies or fractures.

**10:58 a.m.**

Device check. Pacemaker interrogation (gl). Marcus reviews the data carefully. Subtle changes matter here.

He flags Dr. Singh.

"Rate response looks off."

Dr. Singh reviews. "Good catch. Let's adjust."

Small changes. Big downstream impact.

**12:07 p.m.**

Lunch is a sandwich eaten while reviewing labs. Potassium (gl) borderline. Kidney function drifting. Marcus adjusts the plan and documents clearly — cardiology documentation must defend decisions months later.

**01:02 p.m.**

Post-hospital discharge visit. The patient looks scared. They always do after a cardiac admission.

Marcus reviews the hospitalization step-by-step, translating ICU language into something survivable. Med reconciliation (gl) takes time. Time well spent.

**02:26 p.m.**

Another Holter review. This one benign. Marcus messages reassurance instead of scheduling an unnecessary visit.

Knowing when *not* to escalate is part of the job.

**03:18 p.m.**

Shortness of breath visit. Not cardiac. Marcus recognizes it quickly — anemia (gl), not heart failure.

He explains. Orders labs. Coordinates with primary care. Cardiology doesn't own everything, and pretending otherwise erodes credibility.

**04:11 p.m.**

Last patient. Long-term follow-up. Ten years now. Marcus knows the family history without looking.

They talk about travel plans and medication timing. This is continuity most specialties never see.

**04:47 p.m.**

Notes closed. Inbox cleared. Marcus double-checks tomorrow's stress test list.

Dr. Singh stops by. "Good work today."

It's understated. It lands.

**05:13 p.m.**

Drive home. The mental load releases slowly. Cardiology doesn't spike adrenaline; it applies steady pressure.

**05:36 p.m.**

Home. Nova greets Marcus with controlled enthusiasm — tail wagging, posture alert. Dinner is simple, eaten sitting down.

**09:02 p.m.**

Marcus sets out tomorrow's scrubs. Another clinic day. Different numbers. Same stakes.

In bed, he thinks:

*I like that this work rewards precision and patience. I don't love how unforgiving the margins can be.*

The alarm is already set for tomorrow.

Chapter 25

# Day In The Life -- Oncology

**05:22 a.m.**

The morning starts quietly, the way oncology mornings usually do — not peaceful, just respectful.

Daniel Kim, PA-C sits at the kitchen table with a mug of coffee cooling faster than he drinks it. Outside, the sky is still deciding whether it wants to become day. Inside, a golden retriever named Luna rests her head against his knee, sensing the slow weight of the specialty her owner chose years ago.

Daniel is a **career Medical Oncology Physician Assistant**, nine years into practice, working in a combined outpatient infusion and oncology clinic attached to a regional cancer center. He didn't land here by accident. Early in his training, he realized he was less drawn to fast decisions and more drawn to long journeys — the kind where patients come back again and again, sometimes for years.

**05:47 a.m.**

Breakfast is oatmeal and berries eaten deliberately. Oncology days require steadiness. Scrubs pressed. Badge clipped. Phone checked for overnight lab alerts — neutropenia (gl) flagged on one patient, mild but worth attention.

**06:31 a.m.**

The drive in is quiet. Daniel reviews names, not diagnoses. In oncology, remembering who someone is matters as much as what they have.

**07:04 a.m.**

Clinic opens. Infusion chairs already filling. The atmosphere is calm in a way outsiders often misunderstand — not because things are easy, but because everyone here understands the stakes.

Dr. Alvarez, MD — supervising oncologist — is reviewing imaging reports in her office. She and Daniel have worked together for nearly a decade.

"Morning," she says.

"Morning. I want to review the scan on Mr. Carter before his visit."

She nods. "I was thinking the same."

That kind of alignment is what makes oncology survivable for clinicians.

**07:42 a.m.**

First patient. Follow-up during active chemotherapy (gl). Fatigue worse this cycle. Appetite low. Daniel reviews labs, adjusts supportive medications, and explains what to expect next week — clearly, honestly, without pretending the process is comfortable.

The patient jokes weakly. Humor is a coping mechanism here; Daniel meets it gently.

**08:58 a.m.**

Scan review appointment. Daniel and Dr. Alvarez enter together. Results stable — no progression.

The relief in the room is visible. Daniel pauses to let it land before discussing the next steps. Oncology teaches patience in delivering good news too.

**10:13 a.m.**

New diagnosis consult. The room feels heavier before Daniel even sits down. The patient's spouse holds a notebook already filled with questions.

Daniel explains staging (gl), treatment pathways, timelines. He watches their faces carefully, slowing when confusion appears. Information is only useful if it's absorbed.

**11:41 a.m.**

Infusion floor check-in. A patient feeling dizzy mid-treatment. Daniel assesses, adjusts hydration orders, reassures the nursing staff and patient simultaneously. Most oncology work is small stabilizations repeated dozens of times.

**12:27 p.m.**

Lunch happens briefly — soup and a protein bar eaten at the workstation while reviewing tumor marker (gl) trends. Oncology rarely allows long uninterrupted breaks, but the pace is different from emergency care; it's steady, continuous.

**01:16 p.m.**

Long-term survivor follow-up. Five years post-treatment. Clear scans. The visit includes laughter — something Daniel never takes for granted.

**02:38 p.m.**

Hard visit. Disease progression confirmed. Daniel sits with the patient and family, speaking carefully but directly. Dr. Alvarez joins midway to discuss next-line therapy options. The conversation is measured, compassionate, grounded.

No one rushes out of the room afterward.

**04:02 p.m.**

Documentation, medication authorizations, coordination with radiation oncology. Cancer care is logistics as much as medicine.

**04:47 p.m.**

Last infusion patient checked. Side effects manageable. Next cycle scheduled.

Dr. Alvarez passes Daniel in the hallway. "Long day," she says.

Daniel nods. "Some good news in there too."

"That's what keeps us here."

**05:23 p.m.**

Drive home. Daniel doesn't turn on music immediately. Some days need silence first.

**05:49 p.m.**

Luna greets him at the door with full-body enthusiasm, the kind that resets perspective quickly. Dinner is simple. Conversation light.

Later, sitting quietly on the couch, Daniel reflects:

*In oncology, victories aren't always loud. Sometimes they're measured in extra months, stable scans, or the simple fact that someone made it through another treatment cycle.*

He leans back, the day still present but no longer overwhelming, knowing tomorrow will bring another set of stories — different patients, different outcomes, the same commitment to walk beside them wherever the road leads.

Chapter 26

# Student Success Stories™ —

Before questions get answered, it helps to see how real people arrive here.

Not the polished version. Not the résumé summary. But the winding paths, the doubts carried quietly, the pivots made when reality didn't match expectation. These stories aren't examples to imitate. They're mirrors — fragments of truth that help you recognize what resonates, what doesn't, and why.

Each journey below reflects a different starting point, a different set of constraints, and a different relationship with responsibility. Some arrived in PA practice with certainty. Others arrived sideways, after ruling things out. A few are still negotiating their place inside the role.

None of them are presented as "success" because they stayed.

They're here because they noticed alignment — or misalignment — early enough to respond honestly.

### *Journey One —*

### *The Career Changer Who Needed the Middle Ground*

She didn't come to healthcare young.

By the time she started prerequisites, she'd already built a life in another field — deadlines, client expectations, performance metrics that rewarded output but ignored meaning. The work paid well. It never felt right.

She was drawn to medicine for the same reason she left her first career: she wanted work that mattered beyond deliverables. But becoming a physician felt misaligned in a different way. The length of training. The all-consuming identity. The sense that life would have to wait indefinitely.

PA practice appeared as a middle ground.

Enough depth to engage her intellect. Enough responsibility to feel useful. Enough flexibility to imagine a life alongside the work. She moved through school quickly, fueled by purpose and momentum.

The first job was harder than expected.

Not clinically — she handled that. But emotionally. The transition from autonomy in her previous career to layered supervision felt jarring. She questioned herself more than she anticipated. She wondered whether she had misjudged what "middle ground" actually meant.

What steadied her wasn't certainty.

It was fit recognition.

She realized she valued collaboration more than control. That shared decision-making felt supportive, not limiting. That the PA role allowed her to engage deeply without carrying the entire system alone.

Five years in, she doesn't romanticize the work.

She still notices the toll. She still sets boundaries deliberately. But the role fits the way she wants to live — and that alignment, not passion, is what keeps her here.

***Journey Two —***

***The Clinician Who Wanted the Next Layer***

He came in through experience.

Years as a medical assistant. Then a technician role that put him close to care but just outside decision-making. He knew the flow of clinics, the personalities of providers, the unspoken rhythms of patient care.

What he wanted wasn't escape.

It was depth.

PA school was a stretch — academically and financially — but it felt like a natural progression. He didn't chase prestige. He chased the ability to think clinically, to own decisions instead of executing them.

The reality surprised him.

Responsibility arrived faster than confidence. The transition from knowing *what* to do to deciding *why* to do it was heavier than he expected. He missed the clarity of task-based roles during his first year.

What changed wasn't the job.

It was his tolerance for uncertainty.

As his experience grew, so did his comfort with not having perfect answers. He learned when to lean in and when to consult. The PA role began to feel less like a stretch and more like a platform.

He doesn't need to be at the top.

He needs to be *in* the work — thinking, adjusting, contributing meaningfully without losing himself to it.

***Journey Three —***

***The High Achiever Who Had to Slow Down***

She excelled at school.

Top grades. Strong evaluations. Praise for her clinical reasoning. PA practice seemed like the logical next step — a role that rewarded competence and momentum.

The problem wasn't performance.

It was pace.

She entered a fast-moving specialty and quickly became indispensable. The validation felt good — until it didn't. Long days blurred together. Recovery time shrank. The part of her that once thrived on challenge began to feel constantly braced.

Nothing was "wrong" enough to justify leaving.

That made it harder.

What finally shifted was honesty.

She recognized that her identity wasn't built to live in perpetual acceleration. She didn't fail at the role. The role simply asked her to be someone she wasn't, every day.

Her pivot wasn't dramatic.

A different setting. A narrower scope. Fewer adrenaline spikes. The work still matters — but now it fits the pace she can sustain.

**These stories aren't conclusions.**

They're context.

As you read the ones that follow, don't ask whether you'd make the same choices. Ask whether you recognize the pressures, the tradeoffs, and the moments where alignment quietly revealed itself.

That recognition is where clarity begins.

Chapter 27

# Mini SCRUBfit™ Healthcare Career Assessment

## Physician Assistant (PA) Edition

### Introduction

Becoming a Physician Assistant is not only about clinical ability — it is about alignment with the pace, responsibility, communication demands, and collaborative nature of the role. This brief assessment is designed to help you reflect on how well the realities of PA practice match how you naturally think, work, and operate day-to-day. It is not a test of intelligence or capability. Instead, it is a mirror designed to help you evaluate role fit.

### Instructions

Read each statement carefully and rate how true it feels for you using the scale below.

### Rating Scale

1 — Strongly Disagree

2 — Disagree

3 — Slightly Disagree

4 — Neutral

5 — Slightly Agree

6 — Agree

7 — Strongly Agree

8 — Very Strongly Agree

9 — Almost Completely True

10 — Completely True

Answer honestly based on who you are now — not who you think you "should" be.

**Assessment Statements**

1 I am comfortable making clinical decisions while collaborating closely with a supervising physician.

2 I enjoy working in fast-moving environments where priorities shift quickly.

3 I am energized by evaluating a wide variety of patient conditions rather than focusing on only one narrow specialty.

4 I am comfortable balancing autonomy with shared responsibility in patient care decisions.

5 I adapt well when treatment plans change based on new information or physician consultation.

6 I am willing to carry significant documentation responsibilities alongside clinical work.

7 I handle clinical uncertainty without becoming paralyzed by the fear of making the wrong call.

8 I enjoy explaining medical information clearly to patients and families.

9 I am comfortable working rotating schedules, including evenings, weekends, or high-volume clinic days.

10 I value teamwork highly and prefer collaborative practice environments over fully independent practice.

11 I am comfortable performing procedures when properly trained and credentialed.

12 I can maintain emotional steadiness when caring for patients experiencing pain, crisis, or serious illness.

13 I enjoy learning continuously and adapting to evolving medical protocols and guidelines.

14 I am comfortable being accountable for patient outcomes while working within a physician-led care model.

15 I can sustain focus and performance during long, demanding clinical shifts.

**Scoring**

Add your scores from all 15 questions.

**Possible range:** 15 - 150

**Interpretation Guide**

**120–150 — Strong Alignment Zone**

Your preferences and work style closely match the real-world structure of Physician Assistant practice. This role is likely to feel sustainable and energizing over time if the environment is supportive.

**90–119 — Partial Alignment Zone**

Many aspects of the PA role may fit you well, but certain elements — pace, schedule demands, documentation load, or collaborative decision-making structure — may require intentional coping strategies or careful workplace selection.

**Below 90 — Potential Misalignment Zone**

The Physician Assistant role may conflict with how you naturally prefer to work. This does not mean you cannot succeed; it suggests exploring specialties, alternative clinical roles, or healthcare careers that may better match your operating style could be valuable.

**Closing Reflection**

Career success in healthcare is not determined only by whether you *can* do the work — but whether the daily realities of the role match how you are wired to function. Use this reflection as one data point in your decision-making process, alongside shadowing experiences, conversations with practicing Physician Assistants, and deeper exploration of specialty-specific practice environments.

## Chapter 28

# The 101™ —

These are not test questions.

They are decision questions.

They're the things people ask quietly — late at night, mid-semester, mid-career, or mid-burnout — when momentum has already started pulling them forward. Most Physician Assistants encounter these questions out of order, over time, often after commitments have been made.

Here, they're placed where they belong: **before** certainty hardens.

Read them slowly. Skip around. Return to the ones that bother you. Discomfort isn't a warning sign — repetition is.

***1. Why do people actually choose the Physician Assistant path?***

Most people don't choose PA because they "don't want to be a doctor." They choose it because they want meaningful clinical responsibility without surrendering their entire life to training.

The role offers depth, patient impact, and collaboration without the singular ownership physicians carry. For many, that balance feels honest. For others, it sounds better in theory than it feels in practice. The reason you're drawn to PA matters more than the fact that you're drawn at all.

### *2. What kind of person tends to thrive as a Physician Assistant?*

People who do well as PAs are comfortable with shared responsibility. They value collaboration over control and are able to hold authority without needing final say in every decision. They tolerate ambiguity reasonably well and don't require constant validation to feel competent. Thriving PAs are often strong communicators who can adapt to different supervising styles. Most importantly, they can separate ego from impact.

### *3. Is becoming a PA about flexibility — or compromise?*

It can be either, depending on the environment and your expectations. In supportive settings, flexibility feels real: varied roles, specialty changes, and schedules that can evolve over time. In less aligned systems, that same flexibility feels like compromise — adjusting constantly to others' preferences and constraints. The role itself isn't the deciding factor. The structure around it is. Confusing the two is a common source of regret.

### *4. How much autonomy do Physician Assistants really have?*

Autonomy in PA practice is situational, not universal. It varies by state law, institution, specialty, supervising physician, and culture. Some PAs practice with significant independence and trust. Others find their scope quietly narrowed despite experience. If autonomy is central to your identity, you need to examine environments carefully — not assume the title guarantees it. Autonomy grows, but not automatically.

### *5. Does the PA role change as you gain experience?*

Yes — but not always in the way people expect. Clinical confidence grows, decision-making sharpens, and efficiency improves with time. What doesn't always change is structure. Responsibility often increases faster than authority. Some PAs find that energizing; others find it frustrating. Longevity in the role depends less on skill growth and more on whether the evolving expectations still align with who you are.

### *6. What surprises most people about PA school once they're in it?*

The pace surprises people more than the content. PA school compresses large amounts of material into short timelines, leaving little room for recovery or hesitation. Many students expect intensity, but not the constant cognitive load. The emotional pressure of high stakes and limited margin for error can be unexpected. Support systems matter more than raw intelligence. The experience is survivable — but rarely gentle.

### *7. How different is PA school from other healthcare training paths?*

PA school is clinically immersive early and relentlessly practical. You're trained to think like a clinician quickly, not gradually. The expectation is synthesis, not memorization alone. Compared to longer training paths, there's less time to explore identity and more pressure to perform. That efficiency is a strength — and a stressor. You need to be ready to commit before clarity fully arrives.

***8. How much does prior healthcare experience really matter?***

It matters — but not always how people expect. Prior experience helps with context, confidence, and communication, especially early on. It does not guarantee academic ease or emotional readiness. Students without experience can succeed, but often face a steeper adjustment curve. Experience is a buffer, not a prerequisite for alignment. What matters most is how you learn under pressure.

***9. Is PA school financially worth it?***

The answer depends on debt, specialty, and long-term expectations. PA salaries can justify the investment, but margins tighten quickly with high tuition or prolonged repayment. Financial stress amplifies misalignment. People who enter the field assuming money will "work itself out" often regret that assumption. Understanding the numbers early is not pessimistic — it's protective.

***10. What do people underestimate about the emotional side of becoming a PA?***

They underestimate how quickly responsibility arrives. You go from student to decision-maker faster than you feel ready for. Imposter syndrome is common, even among strong performers. Emotional resilience becomes as important as clinical knowledge. The work asks you to care — repeatedly — without becoming consumed. That balance is learned, not innate.

***11. How competitive is PA school admission, really?***

PA programs are competitive because demand is high and seats are limited, not because only a narrow type of person can succeed. Strong academics matter, but they're not the whole picture. Programs look closely at maturity, healthcare exposure, and readiness for accelerated training. Many qualified applicants don't get in on the first try. Persistence and realistic self-assessment matter more than perfection.

***12. What role does GPA play compared to real-world experience?***

GPA opens doors, but experience gives context. A strong GPA shows you can handle academic rigor under pressure. Real-world experience shows you understand what patient care actually involves. One rarely replaces the other. Programs want evidence that you can both learn quickly and function responsibly in clinical environments.

***13. Is the PA role respected in real clinical settings?***

Respect is highly variable and deeply local. In aligned environments, PAs are trusted colleagues with clear roles and influence. In poorly aligned ones, respect can feel conditional or fragile. The profession itself isn't the problem. Culture is. You can't assume respect comes with the credential — it's built and supported structurally.

***14. How much does the supervising physician relationship matter?***

It matters more than most people expect. A supportive supervising physician can accelerate confidence, learning, and autonomy. A misaligned one can stall growth and create constant friction. This relationship often shapes job satisfaction more than specialty choice. Choosing environments carefully is critical.

### *15. Do PAs feel "stuck" later in their careers?*

Some do — especially if they expected automatic growth or increasing authority over time. The PA role doesn't inherently ladder the way some people assume. Advancement often requires intentional pivots, added responsibilities, or role changes. Feeling stuck usually reflects unmet expectations, not personal failure. Awareness early helps prevent resentment later.

### *16. How easy is it to change specialties as a PA?*

It's possible, but not frictionless. The generalist foundation of PA training allows movement between specialties. In practice, transitions require humility, retraining, and often temporary pay or status tradeoffs. Some specialties welcome transitions more than others. Flexibility exists — but it's not cost-free.

### *17. What kinds of stress are unique to PA practice?*

One unique stressor is holding responsibility without full control. You're accountable for decisions, yet practice within layered oversight. This can feel supportive or constraining depending on the setting. Another stressor is identity ambiguity — being neither fully independent nor purely assistive. How you relate to that tension matters.

### *18. How does documentation affect daily life as a PA?*

Documentation is not a side task — it's a core part of the job. It consumes time, attention, and emotional energy. Poor systems amplify frustration and extend work beyond scheduled hours. Efficient documentation skills are essential for sustainability. Underestimating this reality leads to early burnout.

***19. Are PA salaries as strong as they appear on paper?***

They can be — but context matters. Salary varies widely by specialty, geography, and setting. Benefits, loan repayment, call expectations, and workload change the real picture. A "good" salary can feel inadequate if the cost is misalignment or constant overload. Money should be evaluated alongside lifestyle and longevity.

***20. How much control do PAs really have over their schedules?***

Schedule control depends more on setting than title. Some roles offer predictable hours and flexibility. Others demand nights, weekends, call, or constant availability. Flexibility often comes with tradeoffs elsewhere. Assuming all PA roles offer work-life balance is a common mistake.

***21. What is the hardest transition point for new PAs?***

The shift from supervised learning to independent judgment is the hardest. Responsibility arrives before confidence fully settles. Many new PAs feel competent one moment and overwhelmed the next. This phase is normal but destabilizing. Support and mentorship during this period are crucial.

***22. How common is burnout among Physician Assistants?***

Burnout exists, but it's not evenly distributed. It's more common in misaligned environments than in the profession itself. Repeated role strain, lack of support, and chronic overload are major drivers. Many PAs don't burn out from caring — they burn out from contradiction. Naming that early changes outcomes.

***23. Do PAs feel satisfied long term in their careers?***

Many do — especially those who choose environments intentionally and adapt over time. Satisfaction correlates more with alignment than with prestige or specialty. PAs who expect the role to evolve automatically often feel disappointed. Those who actively shape their careers report higher longevity and fulfillment.

***24. What personal traits make PA practice harder over time?***

A strong need for control, difficulty tolerating ambiguity, and reliance on external validation can create friction. People who struggle to set boundaries are also at higher risk for depletion. These traits aren't flaws, but they require awareness. Fit improves when self-knowledge grows alongside skill.

***25. What personal traits make PA practice more sustainable?***

Emotional regulation, adaptability, and comfort with collaboration support longevity. PAs who separate identity from title tend to fare better over time. Curiosity, humility, and realistic expectations help navigate inevitable constraints. Sustainability comes from alignment, not endurance.

***26. How much does geography affect PA opportunities?***

Geography shapes scope, autonomy, pay, and job availability more than many expect. State laws, local culture, and regional shortages all matter. Rural and underserved areas often offer broader scope and faster responsibility. Urban markets may be more competitive and specialized. Where you're willing to live directly affects how the role feels.

***27. Are certain PA specialties more sustainable than others?***

Sustainability depends less on specialty and more on environment and expectations. High-acuity roles can be energizing or exhausting depending on support and recovery time. Lower-acuity roles can feel balanced or monotonous depending on personality. No specialty is inherently "safe." Fit is contextual, not categorical.

***28. How much say do PAs have in treatment decisions?***

In aligned settings, PAs contribute meaningfully to treatment plans and are trusted to execute judgment. In misaligned ones, input may be limited despite responsibility. Decision-making authority is often informal rather than written. Observing how disagreements are handled tells you more than job descriptions ever will.

***29. What does "working at the top of your license" actually mean?***

It means different things in different settings. Ideally, it reflects appropriate use of training and judgment without unnecessary restriction. In practice, it's shaped by physician comfort, institutional policy, and liability concerns. Some PAs are underutilized; others are stretched. Clarity matters before accepting a role.

***30. How often do PAs work beyond scheduled hours?***

More often than schedules suggest. Documentation, follow-ups, and unfinished care frequently spill over. Some settings protect time well; others normalize unpaid overage. This hidden labor accumulates quietly. Understanding expectations upfront prevents resentment later.

### *31. Is it realistic to expect work-life balance as a PA?*

It's realistic in some roles, not guaranteed in the profession. Balance is negotiated, not automatic. It depends on boundaries, setting, and season of life. Many PAs achieve balance by choosing intentionally rather than defaulting to availability. Assuming balance arrives on its own leads to disappointment.

### *32. How does PA identity evolve over time?*

Early identity often centers on competence and validation. Later, it shifts toward sustainability and meaning. Many PAs renegotiate how much the role defines them. This evolution is healthy, not a sign of disengagement. Ignoring it creates tension.

### *33. What do PAs most often wish they had known before starting?*

They wish they had understood the emotional toll more clearly. Many underestimate documentation burden and system friction. Others misjudge how supervision will feel long term. Most regret not asking harder questions about culture early. Knowledge wouldn't have stopped them — but it would have prepared them.

### *34. How important is mentorship in PA practice?*

Mentorship is critical, especially in the first years. It accelerates confidence, reduces error, and normalizes uncertainty. Lack of mentorship increases isolation and self-doubt. Formal programs help, but informal access often matters more. You should evaluate mentorship availability like compensation.

***35. Do PAs have viable nonclinical or hybrid career paths?***

Yes, but they require intention. Leadership, education, informatics, consulting, and industry roles exist. Transitions are easier with planning and skill development. These paths aren't automatic exits — they're strategic pivots. Waiting until burnout narrows options.

***36. How does the PA role interact with healthcare systems and policy?***

PAs are affected by policy more than they influence it early on. Scope laws, reimbursement, and organizational rules shape daily work. Over time, some PAs move into roles that affect these systems directly. Understanding this landscape helps contextualize frustration. Systems explain more than individuals.

***37. What role does emotional intelligence play in PA success?***

It plays a central role. Clinical skill opens doors; emotional intelligence keeps them open. Managing conflict, uncertainty, and patient emotion is constant. PAs who develop self-awareness and regulation navigate stress more sustainably. This skill is learnable — and essential.

***38. How do PAs handle mistakes and near-misses?***

Mistakes happen, even in strong systems. Healthy environments treat them as learning opportunities. Unhealthy ones assign blame and silence discussion. How errors are handled affects trust, growth, and morale. This is a critical cultural signal.

***39. Is PA practice emotionally rewarding over time?***

It can be, especially in aligned roles. Reward often comes from competence, relationships, and impact rather than gratitude or praise. Emotional return varies by setting and season. Expecting constant fulfillment is unrealistic. Meaning is quieter and cumulative.

***40. When do doubts about becoming a PA usually surface?***

They often surface during transitions — school, first job, or role changes. Doubt doesn't mean the choice was wrong. It often signals adjustment or misalignment. Avoiding doubt delays clarity. Engaging it thoughtfully creates it.

***41. How much does supervision style affect daily satisfaction?***

Supervision style shapes everything from confidence to stress levels. Supportive supervision fosters growth and trust. Micromanagement erodes autonomy and morale. Absence of supervision can feel empowering or unsafe, depending on experience. The quality of supervision often matters more than its frequency.

***42. What role does trust play in PA practice?***

Trust is foundational. It determines how much autonomy you're given and how mistakes are handled. Trust grows through consistency and communication, not tenure alone. In low-trust environments, even skilled PAs feel constrained. High-trust cultures are protective.

***43. How do PAs navigate disagreements with physicians?***

In healthy settings, disagreement is expected and handled respectfully. Clinical reasoning is discussed, not dismissed. In unhealthy ones, disagreement is perceived as insubordination. How conflict is resolved reveals power dynamics quickly. Observing these interactions matters.

***44. How much variability exists between PA roles with the same title?***

Enormous variability exists. Two PAs with the same title can have vastly different scopes, schedules, and stress levels. Job descriptions rarely capture this. Reality lives in workflow, expectations, and culture. Titles alone are unreliable predictors of fit.

***45. Do PAs feel valued by healthcare organizations?***

Some do, many don't — and it's often inconsistent. Feeling valued is reflected in staffing, support, and inclusion in decisions. Symbolic appreciation without structural backing rings hollow. Value is experienced through action, not words. This distinction becomes clearer over time.

***46. How does productivity pressure affect PA work?***

Productivity pressure shifts focus from care to throughput. It can sharpen efficiency or erode meaning, depending on balance. When metrics dominate, moral distress increases. Sustainable roles acknowledge productivity without letting it define worth. Balance is key.

### *47. What is moral distress in PA practice?*

Moral distress arises when you know what good care looks like but can't deliver it due to constraints. It accumulates quietly. It's often mislabeled as burnout. Addressing it requires structural change, not resilience training. Naming it is the first step.

### *48. How do PAs manage emotional carryover from work?*

Management varies widely. Some debrief with colleagues; others compartmentalize. Without intentional release, emotional residue builds. Healthy practices include boundaries, reflection, and support. Ignoring carryover increases risk of depletion.

### *49. How often do PAs reconsider their career choice?*

More often than people admit. Reconsideration doesn't equal regret. It's often part of growth and reassessment. Those who reflect intentionally make better adjustments. Silence around doubt prolongs dissatisfaction.

### *50. What signals early misalignment in PA roles?*

Persistent dread, irritability, and cognitive fatigue are common signals. Feeling constantly braced or undervalued matters. One bad week isn't misalignment; a pattern is. Paying attention early prevents deeper erosion. Signals deserve respect.

### *51. How much influence do PAs have over workflow design?*

Influence varies by role and culture. Some environments invite input; others resist change. Over time, experienced PAs may shape workflow informally. Formal influence often requires leadership roles. Understanding limits prevents frustration.

### *52. Is continuing education enough to stay engaged long term?*

Education supports competence, not alignment. Learning new skills helps, but it doesn't fix structural mismatch. Engagement comes from fit, autonomy, and meaning. Education is necessary but insufficient on its own.

### *53. How do PAs approach career growth without a clear ladder?*

Growth requires intentional pivots. This may include specialty changes, leadership, teaching, or hybrid roles. Waiting for a ladder leads to stagnation. Designing growth proactively sustains engagement. Ownership matters.

### *54. What role does personal life stage play in PA satisfaction?*

A major one. What fits early may not fit later. Family, health, and priorities evolve. Roles that once energized may later exhaust. Flexibility and honesty enable adaptation.

### *55. How do PAs define success over time?*

Early success often looks like competence and approval. Later, it shifts toward sustainability and balance. Many redefine success quietly. Alignment becomes the metric. This evolution is normal and healthy.

### *71. What is "scope of practice" and why does it matter so much? (gl)*

Scope of practice (gl) defines what you're legally and professionally allowed to do. It's shaped by state law, institutional policy, and supervising agreements. Two PAs with the same training can practice very differently because of scope variation. Misunderstanding scope leads to frustration and risk. Clarity here protects both confidence and patients.

### *72. How do state laws affect PA autonomy? (gl)*

State laws (gl) determine supervision requirements, prescriptive authority, and practice limits. Some states allow broad delegation; others are more restrictive. These differences materially change day-to-day work. Moving states can feel like changing careers. Legal context matters more than reputation.

### *73. What is credentialing, and why does it take so long? (gl)*

Credentialing (gl) is the formal process that verifies training, licensure, and competence before you can practice. It's slow because it involves multiple entities and liability safeguards. Delays are common and financially stressful. Many new PAs underestimate this waiting period. Planning ahead reduces disruption.

### *74. How does reimbursement affect PA utilization? (gl)*

Reimbursement (gl) structures influence how organizations deploy PAs. In some settings, billing rules limit autonomy or task mix. In others, PAs are central to access and revenue. Financial incentives shape roles more than mission statements. Understanding this explains many workflow frustrations.

### *75. What does "incident-to billing" mean, and why do PAs hear about it? (gl)*

Incident-to billing (gl) allows services to be billed under a physician in certain settings. It can increase reimbursement but often restricts autonomy. Some organizations prioritize it heavily. PAs feel its impact without always understanding why. This is a system issue, not a performance one.

### *76. How do productivity metrics influence PA behavior? (gl)*

Productivity metrics (gl) measure volume, not always value. RVUs (gl) and similar systems reward throughput. This can sharpen efficiency or distort priorities. When metrics dominate, moral distress increases. Awareness helps PAs contextualize pressure.

### *77. What is an RVU, really? (gl)*

An RVU (Relative Value Unit) (gl) is a billing metric tied to services provided. It's used to quantify productivity and compensation. RVUs don't measure quality, empathy, or complexity well. They shape expectations quietly. Understanding them prevents misinterpretation of worth.

### *78. How do PAs protect themselves legally? (gl)*

Protection comes through malpractice coverage (gl), documentation, and adherence to scope. Clear communication and consultation are safeguards, not weaknesses. Working outside policy increases risk quickly. Legal awareness supports confidence. Fear decreases with knowledge.

### *79. What role does malpractice insurance play in PA practice? (gl)*

Malpractice insurance (gl) provides financial and legal protection in claims. Coverage varies by employer and policy type. Understanding limits and tail coverage (gl) matters when changing jobs. This is often overlooked until it's urgent. Proactive review is essential.

### *80. How does documentation function as legal protection? (gl)*

Documentation (gl) is both clinical communication and legal record. It explains reasoning, not just actions. Good notes protect judgment under scrutiny. Poor systems increase risk and fatigue. Documentation quality matters more than speed alone.

### *81. What is moral injury, and how is it different from burnout? (gl)*

Moral injury (gl) occurs when system constraints force actions that conflict with values. Burnout describes exhaustion; moral injury explains *why*. Treating moral injury as resilience failure misses the cause. This distinction is critical. Naming it reframes responsibility.

### *82. How do healthcare systems influence individual PA experience? (gl)*

Systems shape workload, pace, and priorities. Policies, incentives, and staffing models matter more than individual intent. Many frustrations are systemic, not personal. Seeing this prevents self-blame. Context restores perspective.

### *83. What does "at-will employment" mean for PAs? (gl)*

At-will employment (gl) allows termination by either party without cause in many states. It increases flexibility but reduces security. Contracts and notice periods matter. Understanding this affects negotiation and planning. Assumptions here are risky.

***84. How do noncompete clauses affect PA mobility? (gl)***

Noncompete clauses (gl) restrict where you can work after leaving a job. Enforceability varies by state. These clauses can limit options unexpectedly. Reviewing them before signing is critical. Mobility is a form of leverage.

***85. What is the biggest system-level misconception PAs internalize?***

Many internalize systemic failures as personal inadequacy. When care feels rushed or constrained, they assume they're falling short. In reality, structures drive behavior. Separating system limits from self-worth is protective. This insight preserves longevity.

***86. How do benefits factor into real compensation for PAs? (gl)***

Benefits (gl) often equal a significant percentage of total compensation. Health insurance, retirement matching, paid time off, and CME allowances materially affect quality of life. A higher salary with weak benefits can cost more long term. Benefits determine sustainability, not prestige. They deserve close scrutiny.

***87. What is CME, and why does it matter beyond licensure? (gl)***

CME (Continuing Medical Education) (gl) maintains competence and confidence. Quality CME supports growth rather than checkbox compliance. Lack of time or funding for CME limits development. Strong support signals organizational investment. CME affects long-term engagement.

***88. How do call requirements quietly change PA roles? (gl)***

Call (gl) adds cognitive and emotional load, even when infrequent. Being "on" changes recovery time and mental space. Call expectations are often underexplained. Understanding frequency, compensation, and backup matters. Hidden call erodes balance.

***89. What does "full-time" actually mean in PA contracts? (gl)***

Full-time (gl) can mean different things across organizations. Some define it by hours, others by productivity. Overtime expectations may be implicit. Clarifying definitions prevents boundary creep. Assumptions here are costly.

***90. How do loan repayment programs affect PA choices? (gl)***

Loan repayment programs (gl) can meaningfully reduce financial strain. They often require service commitments in specific settings. These programs influence specialty and geography decisions. Understanding obligations prevents regret. Financial relief changes career flexibility.

***91. What is the emotional cost of "being needed" in PA roles?***

Being needed feels validating — until it becomes constant. Overreliance increases workload and pressure. It can blur boundaries and delay rest. Being indispensable isn't the same as being valued. Sustainability requires limits.

***92. How do PAs know when they are approaching burnout versus normal fatigue?***

Fatigue resolves with rest; burnout doesn't. Persistent cynicism, detachment, and dread are signals. Loss of meaning matters more than tiredness. Ignoring patterns delays recovery. Early recognition protects careers.

***93. What does career longevity look like for Physician Assistants?***

Longevity is shaped by adaptability. Many PAs change roles, settings, or focus over time. Staying static increases strain. Longevity comes from evolution, not endurance. Movement is healthy.

***94. How do PAs talk honestly about dissatisfaction without fear?***

Safe conversations require trusted peers or mentors. Silence protects systems, not people. Naming dissatisfaction early allows adjustment. Fear thrives in isolation. Dialogue restores agency.

***95. What role does identity play in PA fulfillment?***

When identity is fused with role, stress intensifies. When identity is broader, resilience improves. Fulfillment comes from alignment, not titles. Separating self from role is protective. This shift often comes with maturity.

### *96. How do PAs evaluate whether stress is worth it?*

They assess meaning, recovery, and support. Stress without recovery depletes quickly. Stress with purpose can be tolerable. Worth is personal, not comparative. Honest evaluation prevents quiet erosion.

### *97. What does a "good exit" from a PA role look like?*

A good exit is planned, respectful, and forward-looking. It preserves relationships and reputation. Burning bridges limits future options. Exiting well is a skill. Timing matters.

### *98. How do PAs redefine success later in their careers?*

Success shifts toward sustainability and autonomy. Many value flexibility over advancement. Impact becomes quieter but deeper. Redefinition is normal. Chasing old metrics prolongs dissatisfaction.

### *99. What questions should PAs keep asking themselves over time?*

Is this still aligned? Am I growing or just coping? Do I recover between demands? These questions evolve with life stage. Regular reflection prevents drift. Awareness is protective.

### *100. What is the most overlooked cost of becoming a PA?*

The cumulative emotional load is often underestimated. Small compromises add up. The cost isn't dramatic — it's gradual. Recognizing this early allows intentional design. Ignoring it leads to quiet burnout.

### *101. If I'm being completely honest with myself, should I become a Physician Assistant — or would another path fit me better?*

This is the question most people don't allow themselves to ask until they're already inside the role.

Not because they're careless — but because momentum is powerful. Once you've invested time, money, identity, and effort, it becomes easier to ask *how* to make it work than *whether* it truly fits. Capability takes over. You push forward because you can, not because you should.

Being a Physician Assistant is not just about clinical skill. It's about how you relate to responsibility that is shared but still heavy, autonomy that is real but not absolute, and systems that often constrain the care you want to give. Over time, those dynamics either align with who you are — or quietly grind against you.

Some people are beautifully suited to this role. They thrive in collaboration without needing full control. They find meaning in contributing deeply without carrying the entire structure alone. They can hold ambiguity, manage emotional residue, and adapt as the role evolves across settings and seasons of life.

Others discover something different. Not failure — but friction. A persistent sense that the role asks them to be slightly misaligned every day. That the compromises feel tolerable at first, then heavier over time. That another path — adjacent, parallel, or entirely different — might better match how they're wired, what they value, and how they want to live.

This question isn't asking whether you *can* become a PA.

It's asking whether you want to live the composite day you've just walked through — not once, not occasionally, but repeatedly. Whether the toll feels worth paying. Whether the tradeoffs make sense to you, not just on paper, but in your body and your life.

There is no universally correct answer.

There is only the honest one.

And honesty, at this stage, is not a threat to your future. It's one of the few tools that actually protects it.

If you decide the PA path fits, you'll move forward with clarity instead of momentum alone.

If you decide it doesn't, you've saved yourself years of quiet correction later.

Either way, choosing with your eyes open is not hesitation.

It's alignment.

Chapter 29

# What I Wish I Had Known —

Most people don't wish they hadn't become a Physician Assistant.

What they wish is that they had understood the *shape* of the decision earlier — before momentum took over, before identity attached, before turning back felt expensive.

This section isn't hindsight regret.

It's foresight, borrowed.

These are the things people learn quietly, mid-program or mid-career, when changing course is harder. None of them are meant to scare you. They're meant to replace assumption with clarity.

### *I Wish I Had Known That Wanting PA Doesn't Automatically Mean It's the Right Fit*

Desire is real. So is misalignment.

Many people want the PA role for thoughtful reasons — patient impact, flexibility, collaboration, meaningful work. Wanting it doesn't make the decision wrong. But desire alone doesn't guarantee fit.

What people wish they had known is that *alignment is not confirmed by acceptance letters.* It's revealed over time, through exposure to responsibility, pace, and constraint. Some people discover alignment quickly. Others discover friction just as quickly — and assume it's temporary.

Sometimes it is. Sometimes it isn't.

Knowing that early changes how you interpret discomfort. It turns panic into information.

### *I Wish I Had Known How Little Time There Is to "Figure Yourself Out" During PA School*

PA school is not designed for exploration.

It's efficient by necessity. The curriculum is compressed. The expectations are immediate. You are trained to perform, not to pause. There is very little space to ask, *"Is this who I want to be?"* without feeling like you're falling behind.

Many students expect clarity to arrive as they progress.

What often arrives instead is competence.

You get better at the work faster than you get clearer about fit. That gap surprises people. They wish they had known that uncertainty during training is common — and not a sign they're failing.

Clarity doesn't always arrive on schedule.

### *I Wish I Had Known That Debt Changes How Choices Feel*

On paper, debt is a number.

In real life, it's pressure.

Educational debt narrows perceived options, especially early on. It can push people toward roles they wouldn't otherwise choose, or keep them in settings that don't fit longer than they intended. This doesn't make them irresponsible. It makes them human.

Many PAs say they wish they had fully understood how debt would interact with autonomy, schedule, and tolerance for misalignment. Not because they would have quit — but because they would have planned differently.

Financial awareness is not negativity.

It's leverage.

### *I Wish I Had Known That Supervision Style Would Matter More Than Specialty*

People often choose specialties carefully and assume supervision will adapt.

In reality, the opposite is often true.

A supportive supervising physician can make a challenging specialty sustainable. A misaligned one can make even a "dream" specialty feel draining. The emotional tone of supervision — trust, availability, respect — shapes daily experience more than procedural mix.

Many PAs wish they had known to evaluate supervision as carefully as salary. Or geography. Or prestige.

This is one of the most common blind spots — and one of the most costly.

***I Wish I Had Known That Burnout Isn't Always Loud***

Burnout is often imagined as collapse.

In reality, it's usually quiet.

It shows up as detachment. Irritability. Loss of curiosity. A sense of "getting through" rather than engaging. Many PAs wish they had known that burnout doesn't always announce itself dramatically — and that waiting for a breaking point is unnecessary.

Early signals are subtle. Patterns matter.

Burnout isn't a personal failure.

It's often a mismatch that went unexamined too long.

***I Wish I Had Known That It's Okay to Outgrow the Role You First Choose***

People expect their first PA role to define them.

It doesn't have to.

Many PAs wish they had known that growth often requires change — not endurance. That outgrowing a role doesn't mean you chose wrong. It means you evolved. Staying static out of loyalty or fear costs more over time than most people anticipate.

The PA profession allows movement — but only if you permit yourself to move.

Permission is internal first.

### *I Wish I Had Known That Alignment Isn't a One-Time Decision*

Choosing PA isn't a finish line.

It's an ongoing negotiation between who you are and what the role asks of you — across settings, seasons, and life stages. What fits at 25 may not fit at 35. What feels tolerable during training may feel different once repetition replaces novelty.

People wish they had known that alignment requires revisiting — not just committing.

That doesn't make the profession unstable.

It makes it human.

This section isn't here to tell you what to do.

It's here to help you enter the next phase with fewer illusions and more agency — so that if you choose the PA path, you do it with clarity instead of momentum alone.

## Chapter 30

# The Hiring System —

Getting hired as a Physician Assistant is not a single event. It's a system. And like most systems in healthcare, it rewards people who understand how it actually works — not how it's described.

Many PAs assume that strong clinical training will naturally translate into good job offers. Sometimes it does. Often, it doesn't. Hiring decisions are shaped by timing, risk tolerance, workflow needs, and internal pressures that have little to do with your GPA or passion for patient care.

This section exists to make those forces visible.

Not to turn you into a marketer. Not to push you into competition. But to help you move through the hiring process with clarity, leverage, and fewer surprises.

### ***SCRUBScript™ — Writing a Resume That Gets You Interviews***

Your resume is not a biography. It's a screening document.

Its job is not to tell your story. Its job is to survive Applicant Tracking Systems (ATS) (gl) and reach a human being who has limited time and specific needs. That reality shapes everything — from formatting to language to what you leave out.

Most PA resumes fail for predictable reasons. They are too long, too vague, or too focused on responsibilities instead of outcomes. They read like job descriptions rather than evidence of readiness. This doesn't mean the candidate is weak. It means the document isn't doing its job.

Effective PA resumes are clean, scannable, and specific. They make it easy for a reviewer to answer one question quickly: *Can this person function safely and efficiently in our environment?*

That requires clarity over creativity.

### *What to Include — and What to Leave Out*

Include information that demonstrates clinical readiness, scope familiarity, and progression. Clinical rotations matter, but how you frame them matters more. Emphasize patient volume, acuity exposure, procedural experience, and team collaboration. Be precise. Numbers carry weight.

Leave out anything that doesn't help a hiring manager assess risk. Excessive detail, unrelated experience, and generic descriptors dilute impact. Your resume should reduce uncertainty, not introduce it.

If a detail doesn't support readiness, it doesn't belong.

### *Formatting That Works With — Not Against — the System*

ATS systems are literal. They don't appreciate creativity. Columns, graphics, and unconventional layouts often break parsing. Simple formatting protects your content.

Use standard section headers. Avoid text boxes. Keep fonts readable and consistent. Save and submit in formats requested. These choices don't make your resume boring — they make it legible.

Legibility gets interviews.

### *New Graduates Versus Experienced PAs*

New graduates often feel pressure to "look experienced." That usually backfires.

Instead, focus on clinical exposure, adaptability, and supervised decision-making. Hiring managers know you're early. What they want to see is self-awareness and readiness to learn within structure.

Experienced PAs should show progression — increased responsibility, efficiency, leadership, or specialization. Repeating early-career language signals stagnation. Your resume should evolve as you do.

### *Intelligent Interviews™ — How Hiring Decisions Actually Get Made*

Interviews are rarely about catching you off guard. They're about assessing fit under uncertainty.

Interviewers are listening for how you think, not just what you know. They want to understand how you handle ambiguity, receive feedback, and recognize limits. Clinical questions often matter less than how you respond when you don't know the answer.

Confidence without humility is risky. Humility without confidence is equally concerning. Balance matters.

### *Questions You Should Ask — Even If They Feel Awkward*

Asking thoughtful questions is not a liability. It's a signal of maturity.

Ask about supervision style, documentation expectations, and how feedback is delivered. Ask how new PAs are supported in the first six to twelve months. Ask what success looks like — and how it's measured.

The answers reveal more than any brochure.

### *Working With Recruiters*

Recruiters are not advocates. They are intermediaries.

Some are thoughtful and helpful. Others are transactional. Their role is to fill positions efficiently. That doesn't make them untrustworthy — it makes them focused.

Be clear about your priorities. Ask direct questions. Don't assume a recruiter understands your best interest better than you do. Use them as a resource, not a compass.

### *Terms of Care™ — Negotiating Without Burning Bridges*

Negotiation is not confrontation. It's clarification.

Everything about a role — salary, schedule, call, CME support, relocation, onboarding — reflects priorities. Negotiation helps align expectations before misalignment becomes expensive.

You don't need to win every point. You need to understand what's flexible and what isn't. Silence benefits the system, not you.

Respectful negotiation builds trust. Avoiding it builds resentment.

***The Must-Have Addendum — Saying Thank You***

A thank-you note is not performative. It's professional.

It signals emotional intelligence, follow-through, and respect for time. In competitive markets, it differentiates you. In close decisions, it matters more than people admit.

Keep it brief. Keep it genuine. Send it promptly.

This system isn't about gaming the process.

It's about entering it informed — so the job you accept supports the career you want to build, not just the offer you were given.

We're still pacing beautifully.

Say **g** when you're ready to continue — or if you want to pause and do a word-count check after this section.

Chapter 31

# Hiring System — 2026 realities, tight spacing, no filler.

***CareerNav™ — Finding Roles That Actually Fit***

Most PA jobs are never truly "open."

They're filled through timing, internal referrals, recruiter shortlists, or quiet outreach long before a posting gains traction. Job boards show availability, not priority. Treat them as signals — not the whole market.

Effective searching is layered. Start with health system career sites to understand demand patterns. Supplement with professional associations and targeted recruiter relationships. Use LinkedIn intentionally — not passively — to observe where PAs are moving, who is hiring repeatedly, and which teams retain staff.

Patterns matter more than volume. Repeated openings in the same role often indicate structural strain.

***Recruiters in 2026 — How to Use Them Without Letting Them Use You (gl)***

Recruiters (gl) operate on incentives. In 2026, speed and placement volume matter more than fit unless you slow the process down deliberately.

Good recruiters clarify expectations early, share realistic details, and respect boundaries. Poor ones oversell, rush decisions, and minimize tradeoffs. Neither is personal. It's structural.

Be explicit about your non-negotiables. Ask how long roles have been open. Ask why the last PA left. If answers feel vague, assume friction exists and investigate further.

Recruiters are tools. You decide how much leverage they have.

### *Intelligent Interviews™ — Reading the Room While You're Being Read*

Interviews assess risk.

Not just whether you can do the work — but whether you'll require disproportionate support, resist structure, or struggle under pressure. Your tone, self-awareness, and response to uncertainty matter as much as clinical knowledge.

When asked clinical questions, explain reasoning rather than racing to conclusions. When you don't know something, say so — then show how you'd find the answer safely. This signals judgment, not weakness.

Pay attention to interruptions, body language, and how disagreement is handled. These moments preview daily life more accurately than prepared answers.

### *The Questions That Change Outcomes*

Ask questions that surface reality.

Ask how onboarding actually works — not how it's supposed to. Ask who you go to when you're unsure. Ask how productivity is measured and how documentation time is protected. Ask what happens when someone struggles.

Avoid hypotheticals. Ask for examples.

If answers feel polished but nonspecific, keep listening.

***Terms of Care™ — Evaluating the Offer as a System (gl)***

An offer is a bundle, not a number.

Salary is one line item. Schedule, call, benefits, CME, documentation expectations, productivity metrics (gl), and exit terms matter just as much. In 2026, many roles quietly shift burden into unpaid labor. You need to see the full picture.

Compare offers using the same criteria every time. Ask what's flexible and what isn't. Clarify expectations in writing. Verbal assurances fade quickly under operational pressure.

Negotiation here isn't adversarial. It's alignment testing.

***Negotiation Without Burning Trust***

You don't need to negotiate everything. You need to negotiate what matters.

State priorities calmly. Ask for clarification rather than demands. Frame requests around sustainability and patient safety. Most organizations expect some negotiation. Those that punish it often signal future rigidity.

If something is non-negotiable for you, say so early. Late surprises damage trust on both sides.

### *Contracts, Clauses, and Quiet Risks (gl)*

Review contracts carefully.

Noncompete clauses (gl), at-will employment (gl), notice periods, and termination language shape your future mobility. In 2026, enforcement varies widely by state. Don't assume protections that aren't written.

If you don't understand a clause, get help. This is not a place for optimism.

### *Onboarding — The First 90 Days Matter More Than You Think (gl)*

Onboarding (gl) predicts retention.

Strong onboarding includes protected learning time, clear supervision, and gradual responsibility. Weak onboarding throws you into volume and calls it confidence-building.

Ask what the first 30, 60, and 90 days look like. Ask how success is evaluated early. Ask how feedback is delivered. These answers tell you whether growth is expected — or survival is.

### *The Quiet Red Flags*

Pay attention when timelines feel rushed, questions feel unwelcome, or expectations are unclear. Pay attention when turnover is normalized. Pay attention when boundaries are dismissed as "part of healthcare."

None of these mean you should walk away automatically.

They mean you should slow down.

### *Accepting With Intention*

Accepting a role isn't the end of the process. It's the beginning of alignment in practice.

Clarify expectations before day one. Save agreements in writing. Protect recovery time early. Patterns established in the first months often persist.

Choosing intentionally doesn't guarantee ease.

It dramatically improves odds.

Chapter 32

# The 91-Day Pathway™ —

The first ninety days are provisional.

You're learning, adapting, absorbing. You're being watched — not suspiciously, but attentively. How you think. How you ask questions. How you recover from mistakes. How you carry responsibility when no one is prompting you.

Then Day 91 arrives.

And something important shifts.

You're no longer "new."

You're no longer being buffered.

You're no longer evaluated for *potential.*

You're official.

This pathway exists to make sure that moment works **for you**, not just for the system.

***Days 1–30 — Orientation, Not Proof***

The first month is about learning how the environment actually works.

Not the policies. Not the handbook. The lived reality. Who answers questions without judgment. Where decisions really get made. How documentation actually flows. What "support" looks like when the department is busy.

Your job in this phase is not speed.

It's signal detection.

Take notes. Ask clarifying questions. Watch how people handle uncertainty. Pay attention to what's said — and what isn't. Early overconfidence creates invisible risk. Early curiosity builds trust.

You are not behind in this phase.

You are calibrating.

***Days 31–60 — Controlled Independence***

This is when responsibility expands faster than comfort.

You're given more room. Fewer check-ins. More assumptions about what you "should know by now." This is where many PAs struggle silently — not because they're unprepared, but because expectations are rarely stated clearly.

This is the phase to:

- clarify decision thresholds
- confirm supervision boundaries

- ask for feedback explicitly
- correct small misunderstandings before they harden

Silence here is not strength.

Communication is.

If something feels unclear now, it will feel heavier later.

***Days 61–90 — Pattern Lock-In***

By the third month, habits solidify.

How late you stay.

How much documentation follows you home.

How often you absorb work that isn't yours.

How available you are — and to whom.

This is the moment to notice whether the role you're performing is the role you were hired for.

Small misalignments at this stage become expectations by default. If something feels unsustainable here, it is not "just an adjustment phase." It's a preview.

You are allowed to recalibrate before Day 91.

***Day 91 — You're Official***

This is the day the system stops cushioning you.

Not because anyone is unkind — but because you've crossed an invisible threshold. You're now counted fully in staffing models, productivity expectations, and coverage plans. You're no longer onboarding.

You're in.

That's why Day 91 matters.

This is the moment to do a deliberate check — not emotionally, but structurally.

***The Day 91 Checklist***

Before you move forward, pause and ask:

- Do I know exactly who to escalate to — and when?
- Are my documentation expectations realistic and sustainable?
- Do I understand how my performance is actually evaluated?
- Are my boundaries respected — or merely tolerated?
- Does this role allow recovery between demands?
- Can I see myself repeating *this* version of the day long term?

If the answers are mostly yes, you're positioned well.

If several answers are no, that doesn't mean failure.

It means information.

***Becoming Official — With Intention***

Day 91 is not a finish line.

It's a handoff — from probation to permanence, from learning to expectation, from flexibility to pattern. Crossing it consciously gives you leverage most people never realize they have.

You don't need everything perfect.

You need clarity.

Because once you're official, changing the terms becomes harder — not impossible, but more expensive.

This pathway exists so that when Day 91 arrives, you step forward aligned — not just employed.

# Chapter 33
# Red Flags by Day 91 —

Red flags aren't dramatic.

They're subtle, repeatable signals that quietly teach you what the system expects — and what it's willing to offload. By Day 91, patterns are no longer accidental. They're instructional.

This list isn't about paranoia.

It's about perception.

### ***Support That Exists Only in Theory***

If supervision was promised but is rarely available, pay attention. If questions are met with impatience or deflection, that's a signal. Support that disappears under pressure is not support. It's marketing.

Early independence should feel scaffolded, not abandoned.

### ***Documentation That Lives Outside the Shift***

If you're routinely finishing notes at home without protection or acknowledgment, notice it. Occasional spillover happens. Chronic spillover is design, not coincidence.

When unpaid cognitive labor is normalized early, it becomes invisible later.

***Shifting Expectations Without Conversation***

If responsibilities expand without discussion, this is role creep. If coverage increases "just for now," and "just for now" repeats, that's precedent-setting.

Silence is often interpreted as consent.

***Praise That Replaces Support***

Compliments without resources are a warning sign. Being told you're "doing great" while still drowning is not reassurance — it's deflection.

Support shows up structurally, not verbally.

***Boundaries That Are Technically Allowed but Practically Punished***

If saying no is met with guilt, withdrawal, or subtle retaliation, boundaries aren't respected. They're tolerated conditionally.

That condition usually expires.

***Turnover That's Explained Away***

If multiple people have left recently and explanations feel vague, incomplete, or dismissive, assume there's more to learn. High turnover always has a reason.

Curiosity here is not disloyalty. It's due diligence.

### *Confusion That Never Resolves*

Early uncertainty is normal. Persistent ambiguity is not. If you're still guessing how decisions are made, who has authority, or how mistakes are handled by Day 91, clarity is not coming on its own.

Ambiguity benefits the system, not the clinician.

### *You're "Needed" in a Way That Doesn't Feel Safe*

If being indispensable means being unprotected, overloaded, or constantly available, that's not value — it's extraction.

Being needed should not require self-erasure.

### *You're Already Talking Yourself Out of Concern*

If you find yourself minimizing discomfort, rationalizing misalignment, or telling yourself to "just get through this part," pause.

Patterns that require constant justification rarely improve without intervention.

### *What to Do If You See Red Flags*

Seeing red flags doesn't automatically mean leaving.

It means slowing down, documenting concerns, asking clarifying questions, and protecting leverage while you have it. Day 91 is the last moment when adjustment costs are lowest.

After that, change is still possible — but it's more expensive.

### *Why This Section Exists*

Most people don't miss red flags.

They reinterpret them.

This section exists to help you notice what you're already seeing — and trust that perception enough to act intentionally, rather than reactively.

Chapter 34

# The 91-Day Page —

Before you let Day 91 pass unnoticed, stop and check this page deliberately. This is not about perfection. It's about confirming that what you are stepping into is something you are actually willing to repeat.

**Clinical Reality**

• I am clear on my scope of practice *in this setting* — not just legally, but operationally.

• I know when I am expected to act independently and when I am expected to escalate.

• I understand how disagreement is handled when my clinical judgment differs from others.

• I feel appropriately supported when cases exceed my comfort or experience level.

**Supervision & Support**

• I know exactly who to go to with questions — and I am comfortable doing so.

• Supervision is available when promised, not just in theory.

• Feedback is given in a way that helps me grow, not guess.

• I do not feel punished for asking questions.

**Workflow & Documentation**

• Documentation expectations are realistic within scheduled hours.

• I understand productivity expectations and how they are measured.

• I am not routinely completing unpaid work to "keep up."

• My current workflow feels sustainable, not just survivable.

**Boundaries & Recovery**

• My schedule allows for recovery between shifts.

• Call expectations are clear and manageable.

• I am not expected to be constantly available by default.

• Saying no, or asking for adjustment, feels professionally acceptable.

**Alignment Check**

• The role I am performing matches the role I accepted.

• Early "temporary" expectations have not quietly become permanent.

• I can imagine doing *this version* of the job repeatedly.

• If nothing changed, I would still choose this role six months from now.

If several of these feel uncertain or untrue, that is not failure.

It is information — and Day 91 is the moment to act on it.

***What to Say to Your Supervisor —***

***The Day 91 Conversation (PA-Specific Script)***

This is not a confrontation.

It's a calibration.

You are not asking for permission.

You are clarifying expectations now that you are officially in the role.

You can say:

"Now that I've crossed the 90-day mark, I wanted to check in intentionally. I feel more settled clinically, and I want to make sure my understanding of expectations aligns with yours going forward."

Pause. Let them respond.

Then:

"I'd love to confirm a few things so I can continue to grow safely and sustainably as a PA here."

**On supervision and escalation**

"Can we clarify when you'd want me to escalate decisions versus manage independently? I want to be sure I'm using my judgment appropriately within our expectations."

**On documentation and productivity**

"I want to check that my documentation pace and productivity expectations are aligned with the role. I'm finding that some work extends beyond scheduled hours, and I'd like to talk through what 'good' looks like here."

**On boundaries and workload**

"As things stabilize, I want to make sure the workload I've taken on reflects the long-term expectation — not just the onboarding phase. Are there areas you see adjusting as I settle fully into the role?"

**On feedback and growth**

"Going forward, what feedback cadence works best for you? I want to be proactive about growth rather than guessing."

Then close with:

"My goal is to be a strong, sustainable PA on this team. I wanted to have this conversation now so we're aligned early rather than correcting later."

***Why This Matters for PAs Specifically***

Physician Assistants often absorb ambiguity quietly.

They carry responsibility early.

They hesitate to recalibrate once they feel "lucky" to be hired.

Day 91 is the last moment where this conversation feels *normal* instead of *reactive*.

Using it doesn't make you difficult.

It makes you professional.

# Chapter 35
# Day 91

***Day 91 — The Line You Didn't Know You Crossed***

Day 91 is not ceremonial.

No one gathers you in a room. No email announces it. No badge changes color. But something fundamental shifts anyway — and if you don't recognize it, the system will define it for you.

This is the day you stop being provisional.

Up until now, mistakes were expected. Questions were forgiven quickly. Extra time was assumed. You were still learning. Still calibrating. Still protected — quietly — by the label *new*.

On Day 91, that buffer disappears.

You are now counted.

Your productivity is real.

Your availability is assumed.

Your boundaries — or lack of them — are now part of the operating model.

From this point forward, the system stops asking what you *might* become and starts responding to who you have already shown yourself to be.

This is not punishment.

It's normalization.

### *What Actually Changes on Day 91*

On Day 91:

- Staffing models quietly include you without adjustment
- Coverage expectations solidify
- Documentation speed is assumed, not supported
- "Just for now" becomes "this is how it works"
- Your yeses become precedents

Nothing dramatic happens — and that's exactly why it matters.

Because what locks in here is not your skill.

It's your **pattern**.

### *Day 91 Is a Claim Point*

Day 91 is the last low-cost moment to say:

"This is working."

or

"This needs to change."

After this point, requests feel heavier. Adjustments feel disruptive. Boundaries feel like negotiations instead of calibrations. The system has already learned how to use you.

That's why Day 91 isn't just a milestone.

It's a claim point.

Either you consciously step into being *official* — or you quietly accept whatever version of the role has formed around you.

***The Day 91 Declaration (Do This On Purpose)***

Before moving forward, take one deliberate pause and name — in writing, even if only to yourself:

- What I am willing to carry
- What I am not willing to normalize
- Where I need support to stay sustainable
- What version of this role I am agreeing to repeat

This is not dramatic.

It's professional.

Because once you are official, the work stops asking who you are — and starts assuming.

***Becoming Official — With Agency***

Day 91 does not decide your future.

But it *does* decide the default.

When you cross it consciously, you enter the role with leverage, clarity, and self-respect intact. When you don't, you often spend years trying to renegotiate patterns you never meant to set.

This pathway exists so that when Day 91 arrives, something *does* happen:

You notice.

And you choose.

Chapter 36

# Money Map —

Money decisions made early tend to echo the longest.

Most people look at PA compensation as a single number — salary. In reality, pay is a system of tradeoffs that affects autonomy, stress, recovery, and future mobility. Two offers with the same salary can produce radically different lives.

This section exists to help you read the *whole* map.

### *Base Salary Is Only the Surface*

Base salary is the most visible component — and often the least informative.

It tells you what the organization is willing to pay *on paper*, not what the role will demand in practice. Salary without context can be misleading, especially in settings where productivity pressure, documentation spillover, or call expectations are heavy.

Ask what the salary assumes about pace, volume, and availability.

### *Total Compensation Is the Real Number (gl)*

Total compensation (gl) includes benefits, time, protection, and support.

Health insurance quality, retirement matching, CME funding (gl), licensure reimbursement, and paid time off materially affect your day-to-day life. A lower salary with strong benefits can outperform a higher salary with weak support over time.

Compensation that protects recovery is often worth more than compensation that maximizes output.

### *Productivity Pay — What It Incentivizes (gl)*

Productivity models (gl) often reward volume over complexity.

RVU-based (gl) compensation can increase income — and pressure. In some roles, productivity incentives align with good care. In others, they quietly push speed at the expense of judgment.

Ask what happens when productivity targets aren't met. The answer tells you who carries the risk.

### *Call Pay and "Invisible Labor" (gl)*

Call (gl) is rarely neutral.

Even compensated call changes how you recover. Being available alters sleep, planning, and mental space. Uncompensated call or informal availability is a red flag, not a perk.

If call exists, clarify frequency, backup, pay, and expectations in writing.

### *Loan Repayment — Relief With Strings (gl)*

Loan repayment programs (gl) can be powerful tools — especially early.

They often come with service commitments, geographic constraints, or role limitations. These tradeoffs aren't bad, but they must be chosen intentionally. Financial relief can expand options later — or narrow them now.

Read the fine print before relief becomes obligation.

***Cost of Living Changes the Math***

Salary doesn't exist in a vacuum.

Housing, commuting, childcare, and taxes shape real income. A higher salary in a high-cost area can feel tighter than a lower salary elsewhere. Geographic flexibility is a form of leverage — if you have it.

Run the numbers honestly.

***The Emotional Cost of "Good Money"***

High pay can normalize high strain.

Many PAs stay in misaligned roles longer because the money feels hard to walk away from. This doesn't make them greedy. It makes them practical — until the emotional cost compounds.

If the role requires constant self-negotiation, the money may not be enough.

***The Sustainability Question***

Before accepting any offer, ask one quiet question:

*What does this pay require of me repeatedly?*

Not at your best.

Not temporarily.

Repeatedly.

Money should support the life you want to live — not require you to trade it away slowly.

### ***Using the Money Map Well***

The goal isn't to earn the most.

It's to earn *enough* in a role you can sustain without resentment, depletion, or constant exit planning. That's where real financial security lives.

Chapter 37

# Money Map — What PA Pay Really Buys You (and What It Quietly Costs)

Money decisions made early echo longer than people expect. Most Physician Assistants are taught to evaluate compensation by salary alone, but pay is a system of tradeoffs that affects autonomy, recovery, stress, and future flexibility. Two roles with the same salary can produce radically different lives. This section exists to help you read the full map instead of one number.

Base salary is only the surface. It reflects what an organization is willing to pay on paper, not what the role will demand in practice. Salary without context hides expectations about pace, volume, documentation, and availability. A strong number can still come with hidden costs. Always ask what the salary assumes about workload.

Total compensation (gl) is the real number. Benefits, time, protection, and support shape daily reality more than base pay alone. Health insurance quality, retirement matching, paid time off, CME funding (gl), and licensure reimbursement materially affect sustainability. A lower salary with strong structural support often outperforms a higher salary that erodes recovery.

Productivity models (gl) deserve careful scrutiny. RVU-based (gl) compensation can increase income but also shift risk onto the clinician. Some systems balance productivity with support. Others quietly reward speed over judgment. Ask what happens when targets aren't met. The answer reveals who absorbs pressure.

Call (gl) changes the math even when it's paid. Being on call alters sleep, planning, and mental bandwidth. Unpaid or informal call is not a perk. It's invisible labor. Frequency, compensation, backup, and expectations should be explicit and written. Ambiguity here always benefits the system.

Loan repayment programs (gl) can offer real relief, especially early in a career. They also carry obligations that shape geography, specialty, and mobility. Relief is powerful when chosen intentionally and constraining when accepted blindly. Always read the exit conditions before committing.

Cost of living reshapes every offer. Housing, taxes, commuting, childcare, and insurance premiums determine what salary actually feels like. A higher salary in a high-cost region can produce less margin than a lower salary elsewhere. Geographic flexibility is leverage if you have it.

There is also an emotional cost to "good money." Higher pay often normalizes higher strain. Many PAs remain in misaligned roles longer because the compensation feels hard to replace. This isn't greed. It's practical pressure. Over time, the emotional toll compounds quietly.

Before accepting any role, ask one sustaining question: *What does this pay require of me repeatedly?* Not temporarily. Not at your best. Repeatedly. Money should support the life you want to live, not require slow self-negotiation.

The goal is not to earn the most. It is to earn enough in a role you can sustain without resentment, depletion, or constant exit planning. That is where real financial security lives.

Chapter 38

# Shortage Signal —

***Shortage Signal —***

***Is There Really a PA Shortage, or Something Else?***

You will hear this phrase often: *"There's a PA shortage."*

It explains long hours. It justifies urgency. It smooths over strain. But like many phrases in healthcare, it hides more than it reveals.

There is demand for Physician Assistants. That part is real. What's less honest is how often the word *shortage* is used to describe problems of retention, distribution, and design — not supply.

Understanding this distinction protects you from misreading opportunity as obligation.

***Where Demand Is Real***

Certain settings consistently need PAs. Primary care, behavioral health, rural medicine, and underserved communities often struggle to recruit and retain clinicians. These roles may offer broader scope, faster responsibility, and meaningful impact. They may also come with fewer resources and higher emotional load.

Demand here reflects access gaps, not failure.

### *Where "Shortage" Really Means Turnover*

In many hospital systems, repeated PA openings signal churn, not scarcity. Positions cycle because expectations are unsustainable, support is thin, or productivity pressure is high. The role isn't unfilled because no one wants it. It's unfilled because people don't stay.

A posting that never disappears is not always opportunity. It's often a warning.

### *Geography Matters More Than Headlines*

PA demand is uneven. Urban markets may feel saturated, especially in desirable specialties. Rural and less flexible regions often feel perpetually understaffed. State laws (gl), scope rules (gl), and reimbursement structures (gl) amplify these differences.

A "national shortage" rarely reflects your local reality.

### *The Flexibility Myth*

PAs are often described as inherently flexible. In practice, flexibility depends on system design, supervision culture, and staffing models. Many roles labeled flexible are actually elastic — stretching clinicians to absorb gaps without adjusting support.

True flexibility expands options. Elasticity just expands load.

### *What Shortage Language Is Often Asking of You*

When organizations invoke shortage language, they may be asking for:

- extra shifts
- faster onboarding
- expanded scope without expanded support
- tolerance for understaffing
- delayed boundaries

None of these are inherently wrong. But they should be chosen, not assumed.

Shortage rhetoric becomes dangerous when it frames self-sacrifice as duty.

### *How to Read Shortage Signals Intelligently*

Ask different questions:

- How long has this role been open?
- Why did the last PA leave?
- How many PAs have stayed longer than three years?
- What changed after the last staffing increase?

Answers here matter more than headlines.

### *Opportunity Versus Extraction*

High demand can be leverage. It can support negotiation, schedule control, loan repayment, and autonomy. Or it can justify overload and silence dissent. The difference is whether demand is paired with investment.

Opportunity grows where support grows. Extraction grows where it doesn't.

***Why This Section Exists***

Shortage narratives can push people to accept roles they wouldn't otherwise choose — out of guilt, urgency, or fear of missing out. This section exists to help you separate need from pressure.

You are not responsible for fixing healthcare by absorbing its gaps.

You are responsible for choosing roles that allow you to practice well and live sustainably.

Chapter 39

# Pivot Playbook —

Very few Physician Assistants stay in the exact role they start in.

This isn't failure. It's reality. The PA profession is built for movement — but only if you recognize pivots as strategy instead of escape. Most dissatisfaction doesn't require abandoning the profession. It requires changing *how* and *where* you practice.

This section exists to make pivots visible before desperation forces them.

### ***The First Pivot: Same Credential, Different Setting***

The most common pivot is environmental.

Many PAs discover that the specialty isn't the problem — the setting is. Academic versus community. Hospital versus outpatient. Private practice versus system-owned clinics.

Pace, support, autonomy, and documentation burden change dramatically across environments.

Before changing specialties, change context.

This pivot preserves clinical identity while reducing friction.

### *The Second Pivot: Specialty Realignment*

Some misalignment is content-based.

Procedural intensity, patient population, acuity, and emotional load vary widely across specialties. What felt energizing during rotations may feel draining over time. Other areas grow on you once confidence replaces novelty.

Specialty pivots are common and legitimate. They require humility, retraining, and sometimes temporary income adjustments. They do not require starting over.

Experience transfers more than people realize.

### *The Third Pivot: Hybrid Roles*

Hybrid roles blend clinical work with something else — education, leadership, quality, informatics, research, or consulting. These roles often emerge organically when a PA becomes "the go-to" person for more than patient care.

Hybrid roles protect longevity by diversifying load.

They are rarely posted. They are built.

If you're already doing unpaid hybrid work, you're piloting a pivot whether you name it or not.

• • •

### *The Fourth Pivot: Reduced Clinical Load*

Not every pivot adds responsibility.

Some subtract it.

Reducing FTE, changing schedules, or shifting to lower-intensity settings can dramatically improve sustainability. This is not stepping back. It's recalibrating.

Many PAs wish they had known earlier that reducing volume is a valid professional choice, not a personal failure.

Longevity often depends on subtraction.

### *The Fifth Pivot: Adjacent Nonclinical Roles*

Some PAs move into roles where clinical thinking still matters, but patient care is no longer central. Education, industry, policy, operations, and health technology all value clinical judgment.

These pivots require translation of skills, not abandonment of identity. They are easier when planned early and harder when rushed.

Burnout narrows options. Planning expands them.

### *What Blocks Pivots*

Most pivots stall for predictable reasons:

- fear of income loss

- fear of appearing inconsistent
- debt pressure
- identity attachment
- lack of visible examples

None of these mean a pivot is wrong. They mean it needs structure.

### *How to Pivot Without Burning Bridges*

Pivots are most successful when they are gradual, transparent, and professional. Maintain relationships. Frame changes around growth and sustainability. Avoid framing moves as escape.

Your reputation travels with you.

### *Why This Matters*

The PA role is not a single decision. It's a platform.

People who thrive long-term treat their careers as adaptive systems, not fixed tracks. They adjust before resentment hardens. They pivot before depletion forces them.

This playbook exists to remind you that alignment is not found once.

It's maintained.

# Chapter 40
# Alignment Check™

***Alignment Check™***

Pause here.

Not because you're unsure. Not because something is wrong. But because decisions made at speed tend to borrow confidence from momentum instead of truth. This chapter exists to interrupt that pattern before it becomes expensive.

Alignment is not about liking the idea of being a Physician Assistant. It's about whether the lived structure of the role fits how you are wired, how you carry responsibility, and what you need to stay whole over time. Capability answers the question *can I do this?* Alignment answers the harder one: *what will this cost me repeatedly?*

You've now seen the role from multiple angles. The daily rhythm. The emotional toll. The systems that shape behavior. The compromises that are rarely named upfront. This is the moment to synthesize, not accumulate. To decide what the information means *for you*.

Most people skip this step. They assume clarity will arrive later. It rarely does.

Alignment is not discovered by accident. It's claimed through honest accounting.

### *Capability Versus Fit*

One of the most common traps in healthcare careers is confusing competence with compatibility. Physician Assistants are trained to be capable under pressure, adaptable across settings, and resilient in uncertainty. Those traits help you succeed. They can also mask misalignment for years.

You can perform well in a role that quietly erodes you. You can receive praise in environments that extract more than they return. You can look successful while feeling persistently braced.

Capability keeps you moving. Fit determines whether movement is sustainable.

Ask yourself whether the strengths that make you good at this work are the same ones that allow you to recover from it. If the answer is no, the role may still be viable—but only with intentional boundaries and structure. Ignoring that gap is how burnout becomes normalized.

### *The Responsibility Question*

Being a PA means carrying real responsibility without absolute authority. For some people, that balance is energizing. For others, it creates chronic friction. Neither reaction is a character flaw. It's an identity signal.

Pay attention to how you respond to shared accountability. Notice whether collaboration feels supportive or constraining. Observe how you handle decisions that matter deeply but ultimately defer upward. Over time, this dynamic either aligns with your temperament or quietly grates against it.

This isn't about ego. It's about how responsibility lives in your body.

If you find yourself craving either more control or less weight, that information matters. Alignment doesn't demand that you love every aspect of the role. It requires that the core structure doesn't fight who you are.

***The Toll Revisited***

Earlier, you met the Toll Booth. Emotional load. Cognitive fatigue. Lifestyle cost. Those weren't abstract concepts. They were previews.

Now ask a more precise question: *Which tolls am I willing to pay repeatedly, and which ones accumulate interest?*

Some tolls feel heavy at first and then stabilize. Others compound quietly. The danger isn't difficulty. It's unexamined repetition. What drains you once may strengthen you over time. What irritates you slightly may become corrosive if ignored.

Re-read your reactions to the Day-in-the-Life sections. Not what impressed you. What stayed with you. What made you tense. What you rationalized away. Those reactions are data.

Your nervous system keeps better records than your résumé.

***Systems Reality***

Alignment is rarely lost because people don't care enough. It's lost because systems constrain care in ways individuals are taught to internalize. Documentation pressure. Productivity metrics. Staffing gaps. Ambiguous supervision. These are not personal shortcomings, but they become personal experiences.

Ask whether you can tolerate systemic friction without turning it inward. Can you name limits without self-blame? Can you distinguish between what you control and what you don't? Can you stay emotionally present without absorbing every failure as your own?

If the answer is consistently no, the issue may not be resilience. It may be fit.

This doesn't mean the PA role is wrong. It means the *context* must be chosen carefully. Alignment is contextual, not categorical.

***Identity and Work***

Over time, healthcare roles tend to merge with identity unless actively separated. Titles become shorthand for worth. Productivity becomes proxy for value. That fusion increases risk.

Ask how much of your identity you expect this role to carry. If being a PA must validate you, the work will eventually feel heavier. If the role is one meaningful expression among others, it is more likely to remain sustainable.

This distinction matters more as careers mature. Early intensity can feel like purpose. Long-term alignment requires room for expansion beyond the role.

You are allowed to be more than excellent at your job.

### *The Repetition Test*

Forget peak moments. Forget worst days. Focus on the composite average.

Can you imagine doing *this version* of the work repeatedly? The pace you've seen. The compromises you've noted. The tradeoffs you've acknowledged. Not forever. Just often enough that it becomes normal.

If the answer is yes—with boundaries, support, and intention—you are likely aligned. If the answer is no, that doesn't demand immediate exit. It demands redesign. Different setting. Different structure. Different load.

Alignment is not binary. It is adjustable—but only if recognized early.

### *Permission to Choose*

Some readers reach this chapter hoping for reassurance. Others hope for relief. What this section offers instead is permission: permission to choose with clarity rather than momentum, permission to pivot without shame, permission to define success on your own terms.

Choosing the PA path with eyes open is strength. Choosing a different path after honest reflection is also strength. What weakens people is deferring the question until exhaustion answers it for them.

There is no universal right decision here. There is only the one that fits *you*.

### *A Final Check*

Before you move forward, answer these privately, without coaching yourself toward optimism:

Do I feel pulled toward this role—or pushed by expectation?

Am I energized by the structure I've seen, or merely impressed by it?

Can I tolerate the compromises without losing myself?

If nothing changed, would I still choose this in a year?

If your answers feel grounded rather than performative, trust them. Alignment does not shout. It settles.

This is the pause most people skip.

Taking it now doesn't slow you down.

It saves you time you can't get back.

Chapter 41

# Student Success Stories™

These are not testimonials.

They are lived pathways — decisions made under pressure, identities tested in real time, and adjustments that didn't look clean while they were happening. Each story reflects a different kind of alignment journey. Not all of them move in straight lines. None of them rely on perfect certainty.

Read these for pattern recognition, not comparison. The details will differ. The questions underneath them will feel familiar.

### ***Story One — The Career-Changer Who Needed Forward Motion***

Alex did not arrive at the PA path early.

By the time the idea surfaced, Alex already had a degree, a job that paid the bills, and a creeping sense of stagnation that was harder to explain than unhappiness. The work was stable.

The feedback was positive. The future was predictable. That predictability was the problem.

What drew Alex toward becoming a PA wasn't prestige or income. It was proximity. To patients. To decision-making. To work that felt consequential in a way spreadsheets never did. Healthcare looked meaningful from the outside — not glamorous, but real. The PA role, specifically, seemed like a way to enter medicine without losing years to training or surrendering life entirely.

That framing mattered. Alex wasn't looking for reinvention. Alex was looking for forward motion.

The first surprise came quickly. Prerequisites reopened an academic identity Alex hadn't visited in years. Science classes were harder than remembered. Studying after work required a level of discipline that clashed with fatigue. For the first time in a long while, effort didn't immediately translate to confidence.

That discomfort triggered doubt. Not about intelligence, but about timing. *Am I too late for this?* The question lingered quietly until a mentor reframed it: late compared to what?

PA school acceptance didn't erase uncertainty. It intensified it. The relief of getting in was followed by the weight of what had just been committed to — debt, time, and an identity shift that felt irreversible. Alex noticed something unsettling during orientation: many classmates sounded certain in ways Alex did not. They spoke about the PA role as a destination. Alex still thought of it as a direction.

That difference created pressure.

During the first months of training, Alex performed well academically but felt emotionally out of sync. The pace was relentless. The focus was clinical, immediate, practical. There was little room to process the internal transition from former career to clinician-in-training. Alex learned quickly that PA school rewards momentum, not reflection.

The turning point came during clinical rotations.

In one setting, Alex felt small and peripheral. Tasks were assigned without explanation. Questions were answered tersely. The work felt transactional. Alex worried this was the profession revealing itself — efficient, detached, tolerable but unfulfilling.

In another setting, everything shifted. A supervising clinician explained reasoning out loud. Patients were treated as whole people. Alex was invited into decisions rather than shielded from them. The work was still hard, but it felt human.

That contrast mattered more than any lecture.

Alex began to understand that alignment wasn't about becoming a PA in the abstract. It was about *how* the role was practiced and *where*. The profession wasn't one thing. It was many environments wearing the same title.

After graduation, Alex chose a role that surprised some peers. It wasn't the highest-paying offer. It wasn't the most prestigious specialty. It was the one with protected onboarding, accessible supervision, and a team that talked openly about limits.

The first year was still hard. Confidence lagged behind responsibility. Documentation spilled into evenings. Doubt resurfaced often. But the doubt was specific now, not existential. It pointed to skills to build, not identities to abandon.

Three years in, Alex doesn't describe the decision to become a PA as "finding a calling." Alex describes it as choosing a platform that allows continued movement — clinical growth, potential pivots, and work that feels aligned often enough to be sustainable.

The lesson Alex shares isn't motivational. It's practical.

You don't need certainty to choose this path. You need honesty about what you're seeking — and flexibility when the role reveals itself differently than imagined. Alignment didn't arrive all at once. It emerged through contrast, reflection, and willingness to choose environment over image.

Alex didn't become a PA to become someone else.

Alex became a PA to keep moving forward — without staying stuck in a life that no longer fit.

### ***Story Two — The High-Achiever Who Learned the Difference Between Endurance and Fit***

Jordan had always been good at hard things.

Not naturally gifted. Not effortlessly brilliant. Just relentlessly capable. Jordan learned early that effort closed gaps and that endurance was a reliable strategy. In school, in work, in life, pushing through produced results. That pattern worked so consistently that it became identity.

When Jordan chose the PA path, it felt like a logical extension of that identity. Medicine was demanding. PA training was intense. Responsibility was real. These weren't deterrents. They were proof points. If something was hard, it must be worth doing.

Jordan entered PA school with confidence earned through experience. The workload was heavy, but familiar. Long hours didn't feel threatening. Stress felt manageable. While classmates struggled emotionally, Jordan focused on execution. Study. Perform. Repeat.

Faculty praised Jordan's reliability. Preceptors trusted Jordan quickly. Feedback was consistently positive. From the outside, everything looked aligned.

From the inside, something felt off.

Not wrong. Not unbearable. Just...tight.

Jordan noticed a pattern during rotations. In high-acuity settings, adrenaline masked discomfort. The pace was fast. Decisions were urgent. There was no time to reflect, which felt oddly relieving. In quieter moments, however, tension crept in. The responsibility lingered after shifts. Cases replayed at night. The mind never fully powered down.

Jordan told no one. This wasn't struggle. This was adjustment. At least, that's how it was framed internally.

After graduation, Jordan accepted a demanding hospital-based role. The offer came quickly. The team was impressed. The compensation reflected the workload. It felt like validation for years of effort.

The first six months went exactly as expected. Long days. High volume. Increasing autonomy. Jordan handled it well.

Better than many peers. Supervisors noticed. More responsibility followed. That felt earned.

What Jordan didn't expect was how little recovery followed success.

Days off were spent catching up, not resetting. Sleep was shallow. Irritability surfaced quietly. Work began to feel like something that had to be survived rather than engaged with. Jordan noticed a growing impatience with inefficiency, with questions, with anything that slowed momentum.

That impatience was new.

The breaking point wasn't dramatic. There was no single bad case or public mistake. It was a Tuesday. A routine shift. Jordan realized, halfway through the day, that the work felt heavy in a way that effort no longer solved.

That realization was unsettling. Effort had always been the answer.

Jordan began to question whether this was burnout or weakness. Whether rest would fix it. Whether everyone felt this way and simply didn't say it. The idea that the role itself might be misaligned felt almost disloyal — to the training, to the team, to the identity Jordan had built.

It took months to name what was actually happening.

Jordan wasn't overwhelmed by difficulty. Jordan was constrained by structure. The constant vigilance. The weight of shared responsibility without meaningful decompression. The expectation of availability that never truly shut off. These weren't problems effort could solve. They were features of the environment.

Once that distinction became clear, something shifted.

Jordan didn't leave the profession. Jordan didn't abandon medicine. Instead, Jordan pivoted deliberately — first to a role with predictable scheduling and lower acuity, then into a hybrid position that blended clinical work with quality improvement. The work was still challenging. Still meaningful. But it no longer required constant endurance to sustain.

Jordan now describes the early years with clarity rather than regret.

Being good at hard things is a strength. But endurance is not the same as alignment. A role that constantly demands resilience without recovery will eventually consume even the most capable people. That doesn't mean you failed the role. It means the role asked you to trade something you didn't realize was non-negotiable.

Jordan didn't stop being a high achiever.

Jordan learned that achievement without fit is just prolonged strain — and that choosing sustainability is not a downgrade. It's a correction.

***Story Three — The First-Generation Student Who Carried More Than a Backpack***

For Maya, becoming a PA was never just a career choice.

It was a promise. To family. To younger siblings. To a version of the future that had been spoken into existence long before Maya fully understood what the role required. No one in Maya's family worked in healthcare. No one had navigated graduate school. What they knew was that becoming a PA meant stability, respect, and a clear way forward.

Maya carried that belief carefully — and heavily.

From the beginning, Maya was diligent. Prerequisites were planned early. Applications were polished meticulously. Rejections were taken personally, even when advisors said not to. Acceptance felt less like celebration and more like relief. The path was real now. There was no room to falter.

PA school was harder than Maya expected, but not for the reasons people warned about. The volume was intense, yes. The pace was unforgiving. But the harder part was cultural. Classmates spoke fluently about medicine in ways Maya didn't yet understand. Some had family members who were clinicians. Others had worked in healthcare for years. Maya learned quickly, but always felt one step behind — not academically, but socially.

That sense of being an outsider never fully left.

Maya compensated by overpreparing. Every assignment was triple-checked. Every exam was studied for as if failure wasn't an option. Asking for help felt risky. Admitting uncertainty felt like confirming a fear that maybe Maya didn't belong here after all.

During rotations, Maya received strong evaluations. Patients connected easily. Preceptors trusted Maya's judgment. On paper, everything was going well. Internally, the pressure never eased. The stakes felt higher than grades or feedback. This wasn't just Maya's future. It was the family's.

That weight followed Maya into the first job.

The offer was in a busy outpatient setting with high demand and limited staffing. It paid well. It was close to home. It felt responsible to accept. Maya told herself that stress was temporary and gratitude was permanent.

The first months were exhausting. Not uniquely so — just persistently. Documentation stretched into evenings. Lunch breaks disappeared. Maya hesitated to speak up, worried that any complaint would sound ungrateful. When supervisors praised Maya's work ethic, it reinforced the pattern. Reliability became expectation.

What Maya didn't realize at first was that carrying responsibility quietly often leads to carrying more of it.

By the end of the first year, Maya felt constantly braced. Not unhappy. Not burned out in the dramatic sense. Just tense, always anticipating the next demand. Family members noticed the change before Maya did. The pride was still there, but so was worry.

The turning point came during a routine follow-up visit. A patient asked Maya a simple question: "Do you like your job?"

Maya paused longer than expected.

The answer wasn't no. But it wasn't yes either. It was something more complicated — a mix of gratitude, obligation, and fatigue. That pause lingered long after the visit ended.

Maya began to reflect differently. Not on whether becoming a PA was the wrong decision, but on whether the way Maya was practicing was sustainable. The issue wasn't medicine. It was silence. The belief that asking for less meant deserving less.

With encouragement from a mentor, Maya eventually moved to a different setting with more support and clearer boundaries. The work was still demanding. The difference was that it allowed Maya to breathe. To rest without guilt. To be competent without being constantly depleted.

Today, Maya talks openly with students about something rarely named: being first-generation doesn't end at acceptance. It continues into how you negotiate, how you advocate, and how you measure worth.

Maya didn't need to prove belonging by enduring more.

Alignment, for Maya, meant learning that success doesn't require suffering — and that carrying less can still mean carrying something meaningful.

***Story Four — The ICU Nurse Who Thought More Authority Would Mean Less Moral Distress***

When Sam decided to become a PA, it wasn't because Sam wanted more medicine.

It was because Sam wanted less helplessness.

Years in the ICU had taught Sam how thin the line is between stability and collapse. Sam could manage drips, ventilators, codes. Sam could anticipate deterioration before monitors screamed. What Sam couldn't do was change the plan. Decisions were made above Sam's head, sometimes thoughtfully, sometimes not. When care felt misaligned with values, Sam absorbed the distress and moved on to the next patient.

Over time, that pattern took a toll.

The PA role looked like an answer. More authority. More voice. A seat closer to decision-making. Sam imagined that stepping into a role with prescribing power and diagnostic responsibility would resolve the moral friction that had accumulated quietly at the bedside.

PA school felt familiar in some ways and jarring in others. Clinically, Sam was comfortable early. Pathophysiology made sense. Acute care felt intuitive. What surprised Sam was how much of the training focused on efficiency within systems rather than questioning them. There was little time to process why certain decisions felt wrong — only how to execute them correctly.

Sam noticed the irony but kept moving.

After graduation, Sam chose a critical care role. It felt like continuity, not change. The learning curve was steep but manageable. The team respected Sam's ICU background. Responsibility expanded quickly. Sam was trusted — and busy.

At first, the authority felt validating. Orders were written instead of suggested. Plans were owned instead of carried out. The shift was real.

So was the disappointment.

Sam realized that proximity to decision-making didn't eliminate moral distress. It relocated it. The same pressures existed — throughput, resource constraints, competing priorities — but now Sam was responsible for navigating them directly. Decisions still had tradeoffs. Patients still suffered within systems that couldn't bend far enough.

The weight felt different, but not lighter.

What Sam hadn't anticipated was how responsibility without systemic leverage can intensify moral strain. Being closer to the problem didn't always mean being closer to the solution.

In some moments, it meant being the one who explained constraints Sam didn't create and couldn't change.

That realization was destabilizing.

Sam questioned the original assumption: that more authority would equal less distress. It didn't. It simply changed the shape of it.

The pivot came gradually. Sam didn't leave acute care immediately. Instead, Sam began seeking roles that balanced responsibility with relationship — fewer high-acuity crises, more longitudinal care, more room to influence upstream decisions. Eventually, Sam transitioned into a role that combined clinical work with quality improvement, focusing on protocols that reduced preventable ICU admissions.

The work felt quieter. Less dramatic. More sustainable.

Sam now speaks candidly with nurses considering the PA path. Not to discourage them — but to recalibrate expectations. Becoming a PA can expand your voice. It does not automatically resolve moral distress. That requires environments that support ethical practice, not just elevated titles.

Sam doesn't regret the transition.

But Sam no longer believes that authority alone fixes what systems break. Alignment, Sam learned, comes from choosing roles where responsibility is paired with realistic influence — and where caring deeply doesn't require carrying everything alone.

***Story Five — The Parent Who Learned That Flexibility Is Not a Promise***

When Taylor chose the PA path, flexibility was the deciding factor.

Taylor didn't imagine an easy career. Taylor imagined an adaptable one. A role that could bend around seasons of life. A profession that allowed movement between settings, schedules, and intensity as priorities changed. Compared to other clinical paths, PA seemed practical, family-aware, and sustainable.

At the time, that mattered more than anything else.

PA school happened alongside pregnancy. Then infancy. Then the constant negotiation between studying and caring that never appears in admissions brochures. Taylor managed it through planning, support, and exhaustion. It was hard, but it felt temporary. The sacrifice had a shape. There was an endpoint.

Graduation felt like relief.

The first job was chosen carefully. Outpatient. Predictable hours. No call. The team talked openly about work-life balance. The salary wasn't the highest, but the promise of stability felt worth it. Taylor accepted with confidence.

The first months were manageable. Busy, but structured. Documentation crept into evenings, but not overwhelmingly. Then staffing shifted. A colleague left. Schedules tightened. "Just for now" entered the vocabulary.

Taylor noticed how quickly flexibility changed form.

Requests were framed as needs. Coverage gaps became shared responsibility. Staying late became normalized. Taylor hesitated to push back, worried about appearing uncommitted or ungrateful. After all, flexibility had been granted once. Asking for it again felt risky.

What Taylor didn't realize was that flexibility offered without protection is conditional.

As workload increased, so did internal conflict. Taylor still loved patient care. Still valued the role. But the margin that made the work sustainable was shrinking. Evenings felt rushed. Days off felt short. Parenting began to feel like a second shift instead of a separate life.

Taylor tried to compensate by becoming more efficient. Better templates. Faster notes. Tighter transitions. It helped — briefly. But efficiency didn't restore the margin that had been quietly reallocated.

The turning point came not at work, but at home.

Taylor missed something small. Ordinary. The kind of moment that usually feels inconsequential until it happens too often. The realization wasn't dramatic. It was precise. The role was no longer flexible in practice, only in theory.

Taylor began asking harder questions. Not angrily. Not defensively. Directly. What flexibility actually existed? What boundaries were respected? What tradeoffs were expected long term? The answers were polite but revealing. The system valued adaptability. It didn't structurally protect it.

That clarity changed everything.

Taylor eventually moved into a role with fewer clinical hours and more predictability, accepting a lower salary in exchange for real margin. The work was still meaningful. The trade felt honest. Flexibility was no longer something Taylor asked for repeatedly. It was built in.

Today, Taylor is careful with language when advising others. The PA role *can* be flexible. It is not automatically so. Flexibility depends on contracts, culture, staffing, and leadership — not job titles.

Taylor didn't fail to manage balance.

Taylor learned that balance must be structurally supported or it becomes another invisible responsibility carried quietly.

Alignment, for Taylor, meant choosing a role where flexibility was not a favor — but a design feature.

***Story Six — The PA Who Thought Burnout Meant Failure***

Chris didn't see it coming.

Not because the signs weren't there, but because none of them matched the version of burnout Chris expected. There was no collapse. No dramatic loss of control. No single moment where everything broke. There was just a gradual narrowing — of patience, of curiosity, of emotional range — that felt subtle enough to ignore.

Chris had wanted to be a PA for a long time. The role made sense. The training fit. The first job landed well. Supportive team. Reasonable schedule. Enough autonomy to feel trusted. Early years were busy but rewarding. Chris felt competent, useful, and respected.

That's why the shift was confusing.

It started with detachment. Patients became tasks to complete rather than people to engage. Documentation felt heavier than it used to. Small inefficiencies triggered outsized frustration. Chris chalked it up to fatigue and pushed through. After all, this was healthcare. Everyone was tired.

What Chris didn't recognize was that endurance had quietly replaced engagement.

Time off didn't restore energy the way it used to. Vacations felt like pauses, not resets. The thought of returning to work produced a low-grade dread that was easy to rationalize but hard to shake. Chris began to wonder if something was wrong internally — motivation, resilience, gratitude.

The idea that the role itself might no longer fit felt unacceptable.

Chris had invested years into becoming a PA. The identity was solid. The external markers of success were intact. Admitting misalignment felt like admitting failure — not just professionally, but personally. So Chris reframed the experience as burnout and assumed the solution was rest.

Rest helped temporarily. The underlying friction remained.

The turning point came during a routine performance review. The feedback was positive. Productivity was strong. No concerns were raised. Chris realized, sitting there, that nothing external was forcing a change — and that made the internal conflict louder, not quieter.

If everything was "fine," why did it feel so wrong?

Chris started paying closer attention. Not to stress levels, but to meaning. What parts of the work still felt alive. What parts felt draining regardless of workload. The pattern became clear. It wasn't patient care itself. It was the accumulation of small compromises — time pressure, limited autonomy, constant cognitive load — that left little room to recover.

Burnout wasn't the cause.

Misalignment was.

Once named, the problem became solvable. Chris didn't leave medicine. Chris didn't abandon the PA role. Instead, Chris redesigned it. Fewer clinical hours. A different setting. More control over schedule. Less volume. The shift felt almost anticlimactic — but the relief was immediate.

Energy returned slowly, then steadily. Curiosity resurfaced. The work felt meaningful again, not because it changed dramatically, but because it fit differently.

Chris now talks openly about this phase, especially with younger PAs. Burnout is often treated as a personal deficiency or a temporary state. In reality, it is frequently a signal that the role, as currently structured, no longer aligns with who you are or what you need.

Chris didn't fail at being a PA.

Chris listened to the signal before it became irreversible.

Alignment, Chris learned, is not about staying enthusiastic forever. It's about noticing when endurance has replaced engagement — and having the courage to change course before exhaustion makes the decision for you.

That completes **Student Success Stories™**.

Six stories. Six distinct alignment patterns. One unifying truth: most people don't need a different profession — they need a role that fits who they've become.

# Chapter 42
# SCRUBScript™

Your résumé is not a story.

It is a screening instrument.

Its only job is to survive the first cut and earn a second look. Not admiration. Not inspiration. Not explanation. In 2026, most PA résumés fail because they are written for people who never actually read them. They describe effort instead of signal, responsibility instead of readiness, and training instead of judgment.

SCRUBScript™ exists to fix that.

This system treats your résumé as a decision tool used by hiring managers who are managing risk, time pressure, and staffing gaps simultaneously. If your résumé does not reduce uncertainty quickly, it is ignored—regardless of how capable you actually are.

### *How Résumés Are Really Read*

Most PA résumés are reviewed in under thirty seconds.

Not because hiring managers are careless, but because volume is high and stakes are real. The initial read answers three questions only:

Can this person function safely in our environment?

Will they require excessive supervision early?

Do they understand the realities of this role?

Everything else is noise.

Your résumé must make competence obvious without explanation. That means specificity, restraint, and discipline. General statements feel safer to write but riskier to read.

### *The One-Page Myth*

Early-career PAs are often told their résumé must be one page. That rule is outdated and misunderstood. The real rule is this: **no wasted space**.

A new graduate résumé is usually one to two pages. An experienced PA résumé may extend to two or three. Length is not the problem. Density is. If every line carries signal, length is tolerated. If lines repeat information or inflate scope, even one page is too long.

Earn every line.

### *Bullet Construction Rules*

Every bullet must answer at least one of the following:

What level of acuity did you manage?

What decisions were you trusted to make?

What volume or complexity did you handle?

How did your role reduce risk, improve flow, or support outcomes?

Weak bullets describe tasks. Strong bullets demonstrate judgment.

Avoid phrases like "responsible for," "assisted with," or "worked closely with." These hide your actual contribution. Replace them with verbs that imply decision-making, prioritization, and accountability.

Compare the difference:

"Responsible for patient care in a busy clinic."

versus

"Managed 18–22 patients per day in a high-volume outpatient clinic, prioritizing acuity, coordinating follow-up, and escalating care appropriately."

Same role. Very different signal.

### *Clinical Rotations — What Actually Matters*

For new graduates, rotations are not a checklist. They are proxies for exposure.

Hiring managers are scanning for pattern recognition: settings, pace, supervision style, and comfort with uncertainty. Listing every task performed dilutes impact. Focus instead on what the rotation demanded of you.

Include:

- setting type and patient volume
- acuity level

- degree of independence
- key decision points
- documentation system exposure

Avoid listing procedures unless they were performed repeatedly and independently under supervision. One-time exposure is not signal.

### *New Graduate Résumé Priorities*

As a new PA, you are not expected to be efficient. You are expected to be safe, teachable, and self-aware.

Your résumé should emphasize:

- structured decision-making
- awareness of limits
- ability to escalate appropriately
- comfort with feedback
- reliability under supervision

Do not attempt to "sound experienced." Hiring managers can detect exaggeration immediately, and it creates distrust. Clarity beats confidence theater.

### *Experienced PA Résumé Evolution*

At two to five years, your résumé must change.

If it still reads like a new graduate document, it signals stagnation. At this stage, hiring managers expect to see progression: faster judgment, broader scope, increased responsibility, or specialization.

This is where outcomes, efficiency, and leadership begin to matter. Not managerial leadership—clinical leadership. Precepting. Workflow improvement. Trusted coverage. Reduced supervision.

If your bullets still describe what you were assigned instead of what you carried, the résumé has not evolved.

### *Metrics Without Self-Sabotage*

Numbers matter, but only when they clarify reality.

Use ranges, not absolutes. Use averages, not peak days. Inflated numbers trigger skepticism. Conservative specificity builds trust.

Good metrics include:

- patients per shift
- acuity mix
- on-call frequency
- panel size
- consult volume

Avoid vanity metrics. Productivity numbers without context can backfire, especially in systems sensitive to liability.

### *Formatting for ATS Survival*

Your résumé must parse cleanly.

That means no tables, no text boxes, no columns, no graphics, and no creative section headers. Fonts should be standard. Headings should be obvious. White space should support scanning, not decoration.

ATS systems do not appreciate elegance. They appreciate legibility.

If your résumé looks impressive but breaks parsing, it will never be read.

***The Language Trap***

Healthcare professionals often understate themselves out of habit. They soften language to avoid appearing arrogant. This is a mistake.

Clear statements of responsibility are not ego. They are professionalism.

At the same time, avoid overclaiming. Phrases like "independently managed complex cases" should be used carefully and only when supervision boundaries support the claim. Overstatement is worse than understatement.

Accuracy builds credibility faster than ambition.

***Common PA Résumé Mistakes***

- Listing duties instead of decisions
- Overloading procedural detail
- Inflating scope subtly
- Hiding supervision context
- Repeating rotation descriptions
- Using generic adjectives instead of specifics

Most of these mistakes come from trying to be impressive. The goal is to be believable.

### *The SCRUBScript™ Standard*

A strong PA résumé does three things simultaneously:

It makes your competence legible.

It reduces perceived risk.

It invites a conversation.

If your résumé accomplishes those goals, it has done its job. If it requires explanation, justification, or verbal clarification, it has failed.

This is not about selling yourself.

It is about being unmistakably readable in a system designed to skim.

Chapter 43

# SCRUBScript™ — Resume Evolution by Career Stage

A PA résumé should not age passively. It must evolve deliberately. When résumés fail after a few years in practice, it's rarely because the PA isn't capable. It's because the document still speaks in an early-career voice while the role now demands evidence of judgment.

Each stage requires a different signal mix. Using the wrong mix creates friction immediately.

***Stage One — Student / New Graduate***

At this stage, your résumé answers one question: *Can you be trained safely?*

Hiring managers expect supervision. What they are assessing instead is awareness, structure, and discipline. The strongest new graduate résumés show restraint. They do not attempt to compress an attending's scope into student language.

Prioritize:

- clarity about training environments
- explicit supervision context
- comfort with uncertainty
- escalation judgment
- documentation exposure

Use phrases that show decision framing, not decision ownership. "Identified concerning findings and escalated appropriately" is stronger than pretending independence that didn't exist.

Avoid stacking rotations unless they differ meaningfully. Redundancy signals padding. Signal variety instead: pace, patient mix, acuity, system exposure.

***Stage Two — Early Practice (1–2 Years)***

This is where many PA résumés stall.

The mistake is staying cautious too long. By now, employers want evidence of transition — from learner to contributor. Your résumé should reflect increasing confidence without crossing into over claim.

At this stage, include:

- independent task ownership within scope
- volume handled consistently
- decreased supervision over time
- reliability during coverage gaps

• early specialization signals

Language should shift from "assisted" to "managed," but always within truthful boundaries. If you still require frequent check-ins, say so indirectly through context rather than omission. Transparency builds trust.

***Stage Three — Established Practice (3–5 Years)***

Here, the résumé must demonstrate pattern mastery.

Hiring managers assume baseline competence. What they're scanning for now is whether you've become easier to work with over time — clinically and operationally. Efficiency, prioritization, and judgment should be visible without being bragged about.

Strong signals include:

• consistent patient volume at sustained acuity

• trusted coverage or expanded scope

• reduced oversight requirements

• mentoring or precepting roles

• workflow or process contributions

If your résumé still lists duties rather than impact at this stage, it reads as underdeveloped. This is where specificity matters most.

***Stage Four — Senior / Specialized Practice***

At this level, your résumé should feel calm.

No urgency. No inflation. Just clarity. You are no longer

proving potential. You are demonstrating reliability. Hiring managers are assessing fit, leadership, and long-term value.

Highlight:

- specialty depth
- decision ownership
- consultation patterns
- system trust
- institutional memory

This is also where non-clinical contributions belong: quality initiatives, protocol development, onboarding support. These signal maturity without removing you from practice.

***ATS Keywords — 2026 Reality***

ATS systems do not understand nuance. They match patterns.

This does not mean keyword stuffing. It means alignment between your language and the language of the role. Titles, specialties, tools, and systems should appear naturally in your document — not hidden or replaced with synonyms.

Use the job posting as a map, not a script. Mirror terminology where accurate. Avoid clever phrasing that obscures meaning. Plain language survives parsing better than creativity.

Remember: ATS systems screen first. Humans judge second.

***Specialty Signal Tuning***

A general résumé is rarely competitive.

You do not need multiple résumés for every job, but you do need intentional tuning. The same experience can be framed differently depending on the setting. Emphasize what matters *there*.

Emergency medicine values triage, pace, and escalation.

Outpatient care values continuity, communication, and documentation.

Surgical settings value preparation, follow-through, and reliability.

Signal alignment early. Make it easy for the reader to imagine you functioning in their environment.

***Quiet Rejection Triggers***

Some résumés fail silently.

Common triggers include:

- vague scope descriptions
- inconsistent timelines
- inflated autonomy language
- missing supervision context
- cluttered formatting
- unexplained role changes

These do not result in feedback. They result in no response. Your goal is to remove reasons to say no, not to force a yes.

***SCRUBScript™ Principle***

A résumé should never ask the reader to imagine your competence.

It should show it — briefly, clearly, and accurately.

If your résumé reads like it is trying to convince, it is already losing. When it reads like a factual summary of a capable professional, it invites trust.

That is the standard.

## Chapter 44

# SCRUBScript™ — Bullet Rewriting Workshop

This is where most résumés either sharpen or collapse.

Weak bullets fail because they describe *presence*. Strong bullets work because they demonstrate *judgment under conditions*. The difference is not vocabulary. It's framing.

Below are common PA résumé bullets rewritten to carry signal without inflation.

***From Tasks to Decisions***

**Before**

- Assisted with patient care in a fast-paced clinic.

This tells the reader nothing about trust, volume, or thinking.

**After**

- Managed daily patient flow in a high-volume outpatient clinic, prioritizing acuity, coordinating diagnostics, and escalating care decisions appropriately.

Same role. Clearer signal. Reduced uncertainty.

***From Exposure to Accountability***

**Before**

- Gained experience in emergency medicine during clinical rotations.

This reads like attendance.

**After**

- Completed emergency medicine rotation in a high-acuity setting, evaluating undifferentiated patients, initiating workups, and presenting assessment and plans under attending supervision.

Now the reader knows *how* you were used.

***From Procedures to Context***

**Before**

- Performed suturing, I&Ds, and splinting.

This invites skepticism unless context is provided.

**After**

- Performed laceration repairs, abscess management, and splinting routinely during emergency medicine rotation, with increasing independence under direct supervision.

The scope is believable because the supervision is explicit.

***From Volume Without Meaning***

**Before**

• Saw up to 30 patients per day.

This raises red flags without explanation.

**After**

• Managed an average of 20–25 patients per shift in a mixed-acuity outpatient setting, balancing efficiency with patient education and follow-up coordination.

The number now supports competence instead of undermining it.

***From Teamwork Clichés***

**Before**

• Worked closely with physicians and nursing staff.

This is assumed.

**After**

• Collaborated with physicians, nursing staff, and ancillary services to coordinate care plans, manage transitions, and address changes in patient status.

Now teamwork has function.

***From Passive to Trusted***

**Before**

• Assisted providers with patient assessments.

**After**

• Conducted initial patient assessments, synthesized findings, and presented recommendations for diagnostic and treatment planning.

This shows contribution without overstating authority.

### *Addressing Supervision Without Weakening Signal*

Many PAs fear that naming supervision makes them look junior. In reality, omission is riskier than transparency.

**Before**

• Independently managed complex medical cases.

This often reads as exaggeration.

**After**

• Managed complex medical cases with attending oversight, demonstrating sound clinical judgment and appropriate escalation of care.

This builds trust instead of suspicion.

### *Documentation as Signal*

Documentation is not filler. It is liability management.

**Before**

• Completed patient documentation in EHR.

**After**

• Documented assessments, plans, and follow-up in Epic, ensuring clarity, compliance, and continuity of care.

Systems matter. Name them.

### *Precepting Without Inflating Leadership*

**Before**

• Helped train new staff.

**After**

• Precepted new PA hires and students, supporting onboarding, clinical reasoning, and workflow integration.

Leadership without theater.

***When to Use Metrics — and When Not To***

Metrics should clarify expectations, not impress.

Use them when they explain pace, responsibility, or complexity. Avoid them when they invite scrutiny without context.

Acceptable:

• average patients per shift

• call frequency

• panel size

• consult volume

Be cautious with raw productivity scores unless they are normalized for setting and acuity.

***Handling Gaps, Pivots, and Nonlinear Paths***

Do not hide gaps. Contextualize them.

A short explanation in the experience section is often enough. Avoid defensive language. State facts cleanly.

Example:

• Took planned leave for family responsibilities; returned to clinical practice in outpatient medicine with full scope and licensure.

This removes speculation without over-explaining.

### ***The Final Read Test***

Before submitting any résumé, do this once:

Read it as if you are tired, busy, and skeptical.

Ask yourself where questions arise.

If a bullet invites doubt, rewrite it.

If a section repeats itself, condense it.

Your résumé should feel calm, factual, and credible. Not eager.

### ***SCRUBScript™ Rule to Lock***

If a bullet cannot be defended out loud in a clinical interview, it does not belong on the page.

This rule prevents exaggeration, protects credibility, and keeps your résumé aligned with who you actually are.

## Chapter 45

# SCRUBScript™ — Bullet Rewriting Workshop (Rewritten in Full-Paragraph Form)

Most PA résumés don't fail because the candidate is weak; they fail because the bullets read like attendance instead of evidence. A hiring manager is not looking for proof that you were present in a clinic or rotation—they're looking for proof that you can think, prioritize, communicate, and manage risk in the real conditions of practice. The fastest way to strengthen a résumé is to convert "task bullets" into "decision bullets," where every line clarifies the context you worked in, the level of responsibility you carried, and the judgment you demonstrated without inflating scope.

A common weak bullet sounds like: "Assisted with patient care in a fast-paced clinic." The problem is that it hides everything that matters—volume, acuity, your role in the decision chain, and whether you can function under pressure without creating risk. A stronger version keeps the claim honest but makes the signal visible: "Managed daily patient flow in a high-volume outpatient clinic, prioritizing acuity, coordinating diagnostics, and escalating care decisions appropriately." Notice what changes: the bullet now communicates operational reality and clinical behavior rather than generic participation, and it does it without pretending you were the final decision-maker.

Rotations are another place where résumés get diluted. "Gained experience in emergency medicine during clinical rotations" reads like a line written to fill space. It doesn't tell the reader how you were used. A stronger rotation bullet anchors setting and function: "Completed an emergency medicine rotation in a high-acuity environment, evaluating undifferentiated patients, initiating workups, and presenting assessment and plans under attending supervision." That single line quietly answers the questions hiring managers care about most: what you saw, what you did, and how safely you were integrated into the team.

Procedures are where credibility often breaks. A bullet like "Performed suturing, I&Ds, and splinting" may be true, but without context it can sound inflated, and hiring managers have learned to be skeptical. The fix is not to remove procedures; it's to contextualize them accurately: "Performed laceration repairs, abscess management, and splinting repeatedly during an emergency medicine rotation, with increasing independence under direct supervision." The phrase "repeatedly" matters, and the supervision language protects credibility. You're not selling yourself short—you're making your claims believable.

Metrics can help or hurt depending on how they are used. "Saw up to 30 patients per day" can trigger doubt because the number is untethered from acuity, setting, and expectations. If you include volume, it should be anchored to reality and paired with what the volume required of you:

"Managed an average of 20–25 patients per shift in a mixed-acuity outpatient setting, balancing efficiency with patient education, follow-up coordination, and appropriate escalation." This kind of bullet doesn't just announce speed; it shows maturity and judgment, which is what most PA roles actually require.

Another résumé trap is teamwork language that sounds polite but empty. "Worked closely with physicians and nursing staff" is assumed in healthcare and tells the reader nothing about how you function. You don't need buzzwords—you need function. A stronger line reads: "Collaborated with physicians, nursing, and ancillary teams to coordinate care plans, manage transitions, and respond to changes in patient status." This version still communicates teamwork, but it also communicates what you contributed to team flow and patient safety.

Many PAs avoid naming supervision because they think it makes them look junior. In reality, omitting supervision context often makes you look unreliable. A statement like "Independently managed complex medical cases" frequently reads as exaggerated, especially early in career, and it forces the reader to decide whether to trust you. A stronger, more credible bullet keeps responsibility intact while clarifying the decision structure: "Managed complex medical cases with attending oversight, demonstrating sound clinical judgment and appropriate escalation." That doesn't weaken you. It signals professionalism and safety, which are the core hiring criteria in most PA settings.

Documentation is another overlooked source of signal. "Completed documentation in EHR" is dead space, but documentation quality is closely tied to risk and workflow. When documentation is included, it should show that you understand its purpose and the system you used: "Documented assessments, plans, and follow-up in Epic, ensuring clarity, compliance, and continuity of care." This doesn't just say you typed notes; it implies you understand why notes matter and how they protect care.

Finally, gaps, pivots, and nonlinear paths should be handled with calm factual clarity, not apology. When you hide a gap, the reader fills it with assumptions. When you overexplain, it reads defensive. A simple line—"Took planned leave for family responsibilities; returned to clinical practice in outpatient medicine with active licensure and full scope"—removes speculation without turning your résumé into a narrative. The goal is always the same: reduce uncertainty quickly.

The SCRUBScript™ standard is simple and strict: if a bullet cannot be defended cleanly out loud in an interview, it does not belong on the page. That rule protects credibility, eliminates inflation, and forces your résumé to become what it needs to be in 2026—a clear, trustworthy snapshot of how you think and function in real clinical conditions.

Chapter 46

# SCRUBScript™ — ATS-Safe Structure & Layout (2026 Standard)

An ATS does not evaluate quality. It evaluates legibility. Its job is not to judge whether you are a good PA, but whether your résumé can be parsed, indexed, and surfaced for a human review. When résumés disappear, it is rarely because the candidate was weak; it is because the document failed mechanically before a human ever saw it.

The structural rule is simple: **clarity beats creativity every time**. Your résumé should look unremarkable to a designer and effortless to a machine. Anything that makes the document visually impressive usually makes it structurally fragile. Columns, tables, text boxes, icons, logos, shading, and embedded graphics are common failure points. They may look clean on your screen and completely disassemble in parsing.

A strong ATS-safe résumé reads top-to-bottom, left-to-right, without interpretation. Standard margins. One column. Conventional section headers. Predictable hierarchy. When in doubt, boring is correct.

Section order matters more than people realize. ATS systems and human reviewers both scan for experience first. Education belongs near the top only for students and new graduates. Once you are practicing, experience leads. Licensure and certifications should be easy to find and clearly labeled, but they do not need visual emphasis beyond clarity. Skills sections should be short, specific, and grounded in reality, not laundry lists designed to capture every keyword imaginable.

Fonts should be unremarkable. Serif or sans-serif is less important than consistency and legibility. Avoid compressed fonts that save space at the cost of readability. White space should guide the eye, not create breathing room. If your résumé looks "airy," it is wasting space you need for signal.

Headers should be literal, not clever. "Professional Experience" parses. "Where I've Made an Impact" does not. The same applies to section titles like "Clinical Journey" or "What I Bring to the Table." These may feel personal, but they introduce friction for both machines and humans. Clarity is not impersonal; it is respectful of the reader's time.

Dates must be unambiguous. Month and year. Consistent formatting. No unexplained overlaps. If something overlaps intentionally, context must be clear in the role description. Unclear timelines create suspicion quickly, and suspicion is rarely resolved in your favor.

File format also matters. PDFs are generally safest, but only if they are text-based, not image-based. If you export from design software or scan a document, you may create a résumé that looks perfect and parses as blank. Before submitting, always copy and paste your résumé into a plain text editor. If it falls apart there, it will fall apart in an ATS.

The guiding principle is this: **your résumé should survive being stripped of formatting and still make sense**. If it does, it will survive most ATS systems in use in 2026.

***SCRUBScript™ — Specialty-Specific Résumé Traps***

Many strong PAs get screened out not because they lack experience, but because their résumé signals the wrong strengths for the setting they're applying to. This is rarely intentional. It happens when candidates reuse a general résumé for environments that prioritize very different risks.

In emergency medicine, the most common trap is overstating independence without clarifying decision support. Emergency departments are acutely sensitive to liability and escalation judgment. Résumés that emphasize speed and volume without mentioning collaboration, consultation, or escalation patterns can quietly alarm reviewers. EM résumés should signal calm triage, prioritization under pressure, and comfort with uncertainty—not heroics.

In outpatient and primary care settings, the opposite problem appears. Résumés often lean too heavily on task lists and patient volume without demonstrating continuity, follow-through, and communication. Hiring managers in these environments want to see evidence of relationship-based care, documentation discipline, and the ability to manage complexity over time, not just per visit.

Surgical and procedural settings have their own trap: listing procedures without showing reliability. Surgeons care deeply about preparation, anticipation, and follow-through. A résumé that lists technical exposure but ignores perioperative coordination, post-op monitoring, and trust-based responsibilities feels incomplete. In these environments, consistency matters more than breadth.

In inpatient medicine, vague scope descriptions are the fastest way to lose credibility. Statements like "managed inpatient care" are too broad to be useful. Hiring managers want to know census size, acuity mix, call structure, and how decisions were shared. Ambiguity reads as avoidance.

The fix is not to rewrite your entire résumé for every job. It is to **re-weight the signal**. The same experience can be framed to highlight what matters most in that environment, without changing the facts. That is not manipulation; it is professional translation.

### *The SCRUBScript™ Structural Rule to Lock*

If your résumé requires explanation to make sense, it is structurally weak. A hiring manager should understand where you've worked, what you've handled, and how you function clinically without asking follow-up questions just to decode the document.

When structure is clean, bullets do the work. When structure is sloppy, even strong bullets get ignored.

This is why SCRUBScript™ treats layout as a safety issue, not an aesthetic one. Your résumé is often your first clinical judgment in the eyes of an employer. Make it read like someone who understands systems, risk, and clarity.

Chapter 47

# SCRUBScript™ — Why Strong PAs Still Don't Get Calls

When capable PAs don't get interviews, the reflex explanation is usually "the market is saturated" or "they must want someone with more experience." Sometimes that's true. Most of the time, it's incomplete. The more common problem is that the résumé does not reduce uncertainty fast enough for the reader who is triaging dozens of applicants under time pressure.

Hiring managers are not comparing candidates side by side in the early stages. They are eliminating risk. Your résumé is not competing against other résumés; it is competing against the option to keep looking. Anything that creates hesitation—even mild hesitation—often results in quiet rejection.

One of the most common failure points is **ambiguous scope**. When a résumé uses broad language like "managed inpatient care" or "provided comprehensive patient management," the reader is forced to guess what that actually means. Guessing is work, and work is what screening systems are designed to avoid. Clarity always outperforms generality. A narrower but precise description builds more confidence than a wide but vague one.

Another frequent issue is **misaligned signal**. A PA applying to an outpatient role with a résumé weighted heavily toward acute care volume may look impressive but still feel risky. The reader is asking, "Will this person tolerate continuity, follow-up, and documentation density?" If the résumé does not answer that question directly, the application stalls. Strength in the wrong direction still creates doubt.

There is also the problem of **frozen résumés**—documents that have not evolved with the PA's actual role. A PA with three or more years of experience whose résumé still reads like a new graduate signals stagnation, even if the work itself has progressed. Hiring managers expect the document to mature as judgment matures. When it doesn't, they assume growth has plateaued.

Formatting failures remain an underappreciated cause of rejection. Résumés that parse poorly or overwhelm the reader visually often never make it past the first screen. This is not a judgment on competence; it is a mechanical failure. Clean structure, consistent headings, and predictable flow create trust before a single bullet is read closely.

Finally, there is the issue of **overcorrection**. Some strong PAs, after hearing years of advice to "sell yourself," inflate language just enough to cross the line from confident to implausible. Hiring managers have learned to read between those lines. When autonomy is overstated or supervision context disappears entirely, credibility drops. Once credibility drops, the résumé is done, regardless of skill.

The key insight is this: résumés rarely fail loudly. They fail quietly, through friction, ambiguity, or misalignment. SCRUBScript™ exists to remove those failure points before they ever appear.

### *SCRUBScript™ — When to Customize and When to Standardize*

Customization is not about rewriting your résumé from scratch for every job. That approach leads to inconsistency and error. Standardization, however, does not mean rigidity. The balance is strategic.

Your **core résumé** should be stable. Structure, formatting, and the majority of bullets should not change from application to application. This protects accuracy and prevents drift. What changes is emphasis. Section order may shift slightly. Certain bullets may move higher or lower depending on relevance. Language may be tuned to mirror terminology used in the job posting, but only when it remains truthful.

The mistake many PAs make is over-customizing early and under-customizing later. Early-career candidates sometimes rewrite aggressively and introduce inconsistencies. More experienced PAs, by contrast, often send the same résumé everywhere, assuming their experience speaks for itself. In reality, relevance speaks louder than volume.

A useful rule is this: if a change improves clarity for *that* reader without distorting reality, it is worth making. If it introduces risk, confusion, or embellishment, it is not.

### *The SCRUBScript™ Resume Test (Final Lock)*

Before sending any résumé, ask yourself three questions, slowly and honestly. Can a hiring manager understand my scope without guessing? Does this document make my level of supervision and responsibility clear without explanation? Does it feel calm, credible, and grounded rather than eager or inflated?

If the answer to any of those is no, revise. Not to add more, but to clarify.

SCRUBScript™ is not about marketing. It is about **legibility in a system designed to skim**. When your résumé reads like a clean clinical note—focused, contextual, and precise—it does exactly what it needs to do.

Chapter 48

# SCRUBScript™ — Writing a Current Resume or C.V.

A Physician Assistant resume is not a biography. It is a clinical positioning document. Hiring leaders are not trying to understand everything you have ever done; they are trying to determine, quickly and confidently, whether you can step into their environment and function safely, efficiently, and collaboratively. The strongest resumes communicate readiness, clarity, and reliability within seconds of being opened.

The first principle of SCRUBScript™ is alignment visibility. Your resume should make it immediately obvious what type of role you fit best. If a hiring manager must read multiple pages to determine your specialty direction, your application will slow down or stall. Early-career PAs should clearly highlight clinical rotations and the environments where they performed strongest. Experienced PAs should position their current specialty, patient population, and operational strengths near the top of the document so reviewers do not need to search for them.

Structure matters more than design. Highly stylized layouts, graphics, multi-column formats, and decorative elements often interfere with applicant tracking systems (ATS) and reduce readability for recruiters reviewing large candidate volumes. A clean, single-column format using consistent headings is the safest and most professional approach. Standard headings typically include Summary, Licensure and Certifications, Clinical Experience, Professional Experience, Education, and Skills. If a section does not directly strengthen your candidacy for the target role, it does not need to appear.

Your professional summary should function as a positioning statement, not a personal introduction. In three to five concise lines, it should answer three questions: What type of PA are you? In what environments have you worked or trained? What operational strengths define how you practice? Statements such as “detail-oriented professional seeking opportunities” add no value. Statements such as “Physician Assistant experienced in high-volume urgent care settings, skilled in rapid patient assessment, procedural support, and collaborative physician consultation” immediately communicate role alignment.

Licensure and certifications must be unmistakably visible. State licenses, national certification, DEA registration where applicable, and life-support credentials should appear prominently near the top of the resume. Recruiters often scan this section first to confirm eligibility before reading further. Missing or unclear licensure information is one of the fastest ways to lose interview opportunities.

Clinical experience descriptions should focus on function, not task lists. Hiring leaders want to know the pace, complexity, and responsibility level of your work. Instead of writing "Responsible for patient care," describe the environment: "Managed 20–25 patients per shift in high-volume emergency department, performed rapid assessments, developed differential diagnoses, collaborated with attending physicians on treatment planning, and completed same-day chart documentation." This communicates both workload and readiness without exaggeration.

For new graduates, clinical rotations serve as your primary experience. Each rotation should list the specialty, setting, and core clinical exposure, followed by brief descriptions that demonstrate participation in workflow. Including details such as patient volume exposure, procedural observation or assistance, and documentation responsibilities helps hiring managers visualize how quickly you may transition into practice.

Quantification strengthens credibility when used honestly. Approximate patient volumes, number of procedures assisted, or documentation expectations provide context for your experience. Precision is less important than transparency. Employers are not expecting perfect numbers; they are assessing whether you understand the operational realities of clinical work.

Skills sections should be selective rather than exhaustive. Listing every software platform or minor training can dilute the impact of your strengths. Focus on clinically relevant competencies, procedural familiarity, documentation systems, and collaboration capabilities that matter to the role you are pursuing. If the position emphasizes procedural care, highlight procedures. If it emphasizes chronic disease management, highlight continuity-care strengths.

A curriculum vitae (C.V.) differs slightly from a resume in academic or research-oriented settings, where teaching roles, publications, presentations, and scholarly activity may require additional sections. However, even in academic medicine, clarity and organization remain essential. A long document that is difficult to navigate reduces impact. Whether submitting a resume or C.V., your reader should always be able to locate licensure, clinical experience, and current role information within seconds.

Before submission, conduct a final readiness review. Confirm that dates are consistent, formatting is uniform, licensure information is current, and specialty alignment is clear. Read the resume once as if you were a hiring manager scanning quickly between meetings. If your clinical identity and role fit are not immediately obvious, refine until they are.

A strong resume does not try to impress by length. It earns attention by clarity, relevance, and truthful representation of how you practice. When written well, SCRUBScript™ becomes more than a document; it becomes a concise professional snapshot that helps the right opportunities recognize you quickly.

Chapter 49

# ApplySmart™ — Submitting With Intention Instead of Hope

Most applications fail long before interviews are scheduled. Not because the candidate is unqualified, but because the application itself is treated as a formality rather than a decision point. ApplySmart™ reframes submission as an active strategy rather than a passive step.

In 2026, applications are filtered by systems, time pressure, and risk aversion. The goal is not to "get noticed." The goal is to **survive screening intact** and reach a human with enough context to say yes.

That requires sequencing, restraint, and preparation—not volume.

### *Why Volume Hurts More Than It Helps*

Submitting dozens of applications indiscriminately feels productive. It rarely is. High-volume application behavior creates two problems. First, it dilutes customization to the point of misalignment. Second, it trains candidates to tolerate silence as normal, which masks feedback signals.

ApplySmart™ favors **selective submission**. Fewer applications. Better alignment. Stronger signal. Each submission should feel intentional enough that you can explain why you applied there and what specifically fits.

If you cannot articulate that internally, the application will not articulate it externally.

### *Application Sequencing — Order Matters*

Not all applications should be submitted at the same time.

Start with roles that are strongest fits, not weakest. Early submissions benefit from focus, energy, and clarity. They also generate feedback—silence, responses, interviews—that informs later applications. Applying everywhere at once eliminates learning.

There is also a timing reality. Many PA roles are posted after internal approval but before staffing urgency peaks. Applying early often means being reviewed calmly. Applying late often means being triaged quickly. Neither is guaranteed, but awareness improves odds.

### *Cover Letters — When They Help and When They Hurt*

Cover letters are optional in theory and decisive in practice. When generic, they hurt more than they help. When specific, they accelerate trust.

A useful cover letter does three things only. It names the role clearly. It explains why the setting makes sense for you. It previews how your experience fits the environment's needs. Anything beyond that is noise.

Do not repeat your résumé. Do not tell your life story. Do not perform enthusiasm. Write as if you are clarifying alignment, not auditioning for approval.

If you cannot be specific about why this role fits, skip the letter entirely.

***The Hidden Application Filter***

Many applications are quietly filtered before clinical leaders ever see them. HR screeners are looking for red flags, not excellence. Gaps without explanation. Inflated scope. Formatting issues. Inconsistent timelines. These trigger rejection even when clinical skill is strong.

ApplySmart™ reduces these risks by ensuring that what you submit matches what the system expects. Clean formatting. Clear scope. Honest progression. Nothing surprising.

Surprise is not your friend at this stage.

***Pre-Interview Intelligence™ — Research That Actually Matters***

Pre-Interview Intelligence™ is not about memorizing mission statements. It is about understanding context. Before any interview, you should know how the organization behaves under pressure, not just how it presents itself.

Start with public signals. Leadership turnover. Recent mergers. Lawsuits. Union activity. Expansion or contraction patterns. These details shape daily practice more than vision statements ever will.

Then move inward. Read job postings carefully. Look for what is emphasized and what is absent. Vague supervision language. Broad scope promises. Repeated mentions of “flexibility” without structure. These patterns are predictive.

Finally, listen to informal sources. Colleagues. Professional forums. Reputation travels fast in healthcare. While anecdotes are imperfect, patterns are rarely accidental.

***Reading Between the Lines***

Every organization tells you who they are if you read carefully.

Frequent reposting of the same role often signals retention problems. Overly aggressive timelines can indicate coverage gaps. Excessive emphasis on culture without operational detail usually means culture is compensating for something else.

None of these automatically disqualify a role. They inform the questions you need to ask later.

***What to Prepare Before the Interview Is Offered***

Waiting for an interview invitation to prepare is a mistake. ApplySmart™ treats preparation as parallel work.

Before interviews, clarify your non-negotiables. Schedule limits. Call tolerance. Supervision needs. Growth expectations. Knowing these in advance prevents reactive decision-making when offers arrive.

Also prepare your narrative. Not a script, but a throughline. Why this role now. What you bring. What you are building toward. When this narrative is clear internally, it comes across as calm confidence rather than performance.

***ApplySmart™ Rule to Lock***

An application should never feel like a message in a bottle. If you cannot describe why you are a fit and what you are testing by applying, you are outsourcing judgment to chance.

ApplySmart™ restores agency to a process designed to feel opaque.

***Pre-Interview Intelligence™ Rule to Lock***

If an organization cannot tolerate thoughtful questions during interviews, it will not tolerate boundaries after hire. Research exists to protect you, not to impress them.

# Chapter 50
# Intelligent Interviews™

Interviews are not evaluations of personality. They are risk assessments conducted under time pressure. Every question —clinical, behavioral, or conversational—is designed to answer one underlying concern: *Can this person function safely and predictably in our environment without creating downstream problems?*

Most PA candidates prepare as if interviews are about impressing. They are not. They are about reducing uncertainty. The candidates who perform best are rarely the most polished speakers; they are the ones who answer precisely, stay inside their scope, and demonstrate judgment without dramatizing it.

Intelligent Interviews™ exists to reframe the process so you stop performing and start signaling.

### *What Interviewers Are Actually Evaluating*

Interviewers are listening for four things simultaneously, even when they don't articulate them clearly: clinical reasoning, self-awareness, reliability, and fit with existing systems.

Technical knowledge matters, but it is rarely the deciding factor. What matters more is how you *think* when you don't know something, how you manage ambiguity, and whether you recognize limits without being prompted.

Strong candidates answer questions in a way that mirrors how they practice. They contextualize. They acknowledge uncertainty. They show escalation pathways. Weak candidates rush to certainty, overextend answers, or try to sound definitive in situations that are inherently gray.

When an interviewer asks about a difficult case, they are not looking for heroics. They are looking for judgment. They want to know what you noticed, what concerned you, what you did first, and who you involved. The safest answers are often the most structured ones.

### *Clinical Questions — How to Answer Without Overreaching*

Clinical interview questions are not board exams. They are simulations of thought process. When asked how you would manage a scenario, resist the urge to sprint to diagnosis or treatment. Instead, slow down deliberately. Start with assessment. Name what you would want to clarify. Identify red flags. Then discuss next steps within your scope.

A common mistake is answering as if you are alone. In real practice, you are rarely alone. Naming consultation, supervision, and collaboration is not a weakness. It is a signal that you understand how care is actually delivered.

Saying "I would discuss this with my supervising physician" does not diminish your competence. It increases it—*if* you also explain what information you would bring to that discussion and why.

***Behavioral Questions — The Trap of Polished Stories***

Behavioral questions are often framed as opportunities to showcase leadership, resilience, or teamwork. In reality, they are tests of pattern recognition. Interviewers are listening for whether your responses reflect insight or rehearsal.

Overly polished stories often backfire. They sound curated. They avoid tension. They resolve too neatly. Real clinical work is messier, and interviewers know that.

The strongest behavioral answers acknowledge complexity. They include moments of uncertainty. They show learning without self-flagellation. Most importantly, they demonstrate that you can reflect on experience without being defensive or performative.

***The "I Don't Know" Moment***

Every good interview includes a moment where you don't know the answer. This is intentional.

What matters is not the gap in knowledge. It is how you handle it. Saying "I don't know" is acceptable only when followed by process. What would you do next? What resources would you consult? Who would you involve? How would you ensure patient safety while clarifying?

Trying to bluff through uncertainty is one of the fastest ways to lose trust. Calm acknowledgment paired with structured thinking builds far more confidence than partial recall delivered with certainty.

### *Panel Interviews vs One-on-One*

Panel interviews are not harder; they are different. They are designed to observe consistency. When multiple people ask variations of the same question, they are watching whether your answers align or drift.

The key is to stay anchored. Do not tailor your answers dramatically to each person. Answer truthfully and consistently. Let alignment do the work. Inconsistent answers create quiet doubt even when each individual answer sounds reasonable.

One-on-one interviews, by contrast, often drift conversationally. The risk here is oversharing. Keep responses grounded. Professional warmth matters more than personal disclosure.

### *Red Flags You Should Notice*

Interviews are not one-directional. Pay attention to what makes you hesitate internally. Vague supervision structures. Dismissive language about workload. Casual references to chronic understaffing. Defensiveness when boundaries are mentioned.

These moments are data, not inconveniences. Intelligent candidates notice them and ask clarifying questions rather than brushing them aside in the moment.

### *Post-Interview Signaling*

What you do after the interview still matters. Thoughtful follow-up is not about gratitude theater. It is about reinforcing professionalism and clarity. A concise thank-you that references a specific aspect of the conversation signals attentiveness and respect. Overly long messages dilute impact.

Silence after an interview is also information. Extended delays often indicate internal uncertainty rather than rejection. Resist the urge to overinterpret or oversell.

***The Intelligent Interviews™ Standard***

A successful interview does not leave the room buzzing. It leaves the room calm. Interviewers should feel that you understand your role, respect systems, and will not create surprises.

That is the goal.

You are not there to convince them you are exceptional. You are there to demonstrate that you are **reliably competent, self-aware, and aligned with the realities of the work**.

That combination is rare—and it is exactly what most teams are looking for.

***Intelligent Interviews™ — Question Patterns You Will Hear (and What They're Really Testing)***

Interview questions rarely change. What changes is how directly they reveal their intent. Once you recognize the pattern behind the question, you stop reacting and start answering strategically.

When an interviewer asks, "Tell me about a difficult case," they are not testing your clinical brilliance. They are testing your relationship to complexity. They want to know whether you notice early warning signs, whether you tolerate uncertainty without freezing or overreaching, and whether you understand when to involve others. The strongest answers describe how the situation unfolded over time, what triggered concern, and how decisions were sequenced. Jumping straight to diagnosis or outcome skips the part they care about most: judgment under evolving conditions.

Questions like "How do you handle stress?" are rarely about stress. They are about predictability. Interviewers are listening for whether you externalize pressure onto others, internalize it silently, or manage it through structure. Answers that focus on generic coping strategies sound hollow. Answers that describe how you adjust workflow, communicate limits, and recover between shifts feel grounded and believable.

"Why do you want to work here?" is another disguised question. The surface answer is interest. The underlying concern is retention. Interviewers want to know whether you understand the reality of the role you're applying for or whether you're projecting an idealized version of it. Specificity matters here. Naming aspects of the setting, patient population, or team structure signals that you've done your homework and that your expectations are anchored in reality.

### *Clinical Scenarios — Showing Judgment Without Playing Doctor*

Clinical scenarios are designed to expose how you think, not how much you know. The safest approach is to narrate your reasoning out loud. Start with assessment. Identify what worries you. Clarify what information you need. Then move into action, always staying inside your scope.

One of the most common missteps is answering as if you are practicing independently when the role does not support that level of autonomy. Another is answering as if you are being tested for speed. Neither is true. Interviewers would rather hear a slower, structured answer that includes consultation than a fast answer that skips safeguards.

If you are unsure, say so calmly and explain how you would close the gap. That response signals maturity. Trying to bluff through uncertainty does the opposite.

### *Behavioral Questions — What Makes Answers Ring True*

Behavioral questions are often framed around conflict, mistakes, or feedback. These questions are not traps, but they do punish rehearsed perfection. Interviewers know when a story has been polished into something frictionless, and frictionless stories rarely reflect real clinical environments.

Strong answers acknowledge tension without dramatizing it. They show learning without self-condemnation. They demonstrate accountability without self-erasure. The goal is not to present yourself as flawless, but as reflective and responsive.

When discussing mistakes, avoid the twin extremes of minimization and overexposure. State what happened, what you learned, and what changed in your practice. That arc is enough. Anything beyond that usually detracts rather than adds.

### *Reading the Room — Interviews as Two-Way Signals*

Intelligent interviewing requires paying attention not just to what is asked, but how it is asked. Tone, pacing, and follow-up questions all convey information about the environment you are entering.

Pay attention to whether questions are curious or interrogative, whether supervision is described clearly or vaguely, and whether workload concerns are acknowledged or brushed aside. These signals matter more than polished mission statements.

If an interviewer struggles to explain onboarding, supervision, or escalation pathways, assume those systems are underdeveloped. That does not mean the job is wrong, but it does mean the burden of clarity may fall on you once hired.

### *Red-Flag Interview Dynamics*

Some red flags are obvious. Many are subtle.

Repeated references to "wearing many hats" without accompanying support structures often signal chronic understaffing. Casual jokes about burnout usually aren't jokes. Defensive responses to questions about boundaries suggest those boundaries are routinely crossed.

Another under-discussed red flag is inconsistency between interviewers. When one person describes autonomy and another describes tight control, the issue is not nuance—it is misalignment. You should notice that tension and clarify it before accepting any offer.

### *Post-Interview Follow-Up — What Actually Matters*

Follow-up communication is not about gratitude performance. It is about reinforcing professionalism and memory. A concise message that references a specific discussion point signals attention and respect. Long, emotional messages often dilute impact and can feel misaligned with clinical culture.

Silence after an interview should be interpreted cautiously. Delays often reflect internal logistics, not candidate quality. Resist the urge to chase reassurance. Calm persistence reads stronger than anxious follow-up.

### ***The Intelligent Interviews™ Rule to Lock***

A good interview does not end with excitement. It ends with clarity. Both sides should leave with a realistic understanding of expectations, support, and fit.

If you walk out feeling relieved rather than exhilarated, that is often a good sign. Relief usually means alignment. Exhilaration without clarity often means projection.

Chapter 51

# Intelligent Interviews™ — Question Patterns You Will Hear (and What They're Really Testing)

**Question Patterns You Will Hear (and What They're Really Testing)**

Physician Assistant interviews rarely revolve around textbook medicine. Most hiring leaders already assume that if you reached the interview stage, you possess the clinical baseline required to perform the job safely. What they are trying to determine instead is whether you can **function inside the real operating conditions of their department** — pace, collaboration expectations, communication style, emotional steadiness, and long-term reliability.

Understanding what interview questions are *actually testing* gives you a powerful advantage. Instead of guessing what the "right answer" might be, you can respond in a way that demonstrates how you think, how you work, and how you operate under pressure.

Below are the most common interview question categories

Physician Assistants encounter, along with the deeper evaluation signal behind each one.

**1. "Tell me about yourself."**

**What they are really testing:** Professional identity clarity and communication structure.

Interviewers are not asking for your life story. They want to see whether you can organize information quickly and present it in a structured, professional way — a skill you will use every day when presenting patient cases.

**Strong response structure**

- Brief professional background
- Clinical training highlights
- Key interests or specialty exposure
- What attracts you to this specific role

A concise, organized answer signals clinical thinking discipline.

**2. "Why did you choose the Physician Assistant profession?"**

**What they are really testing:** Motivation stability.

Healthcare organizations want clinicians who chose the role intentionally, not individuals who arrived by accident or default. They are listening for whether your decision reflects:

- long-term career intent
- understanding of the PA scope

• awareness of the collaborative model

A thoughtful answer shows commitment and lowers perceived turnover risk.

**3. "Describe a difficult patient interaction."**

**What they are really testing:** Emotional regulation and communication maturity.

Clinical ability matters, but patient-facing roles require the ability to remain composed when emotions escalate. Interviewers want to know:

• how you respond under interpersonal stress

• whether you escalate conflict or stabilize it

• how you maintain professionalism during tension

A strong answer emphasizes listening, empathy, boundaries, and resolution.

**4. "Tell us about a mistake you made."**

**What they are really testing:** Accountability and safety culture alignment.

Healthcare organizations value clinicians who acknowledge errors early rather than conceal them. The correct approach is not to claim perfection but to demonstrate:

• ownership

• corrective action

• learning integration

• prevention strategies

This question evaluates whether you will contribute to a culture of safety.

**5. "How do you handle a heavy patient load?"**

**What they are really testing:** Workflow management and endurance.

Departments want to know whether you can:

- prioritize effectively
- maintain accuracy under speed
- communicate when overwhelmed
- ask for help appropriately

Answers should demonstrate both productivity awareness and patient safety balance.

**6. "Describe your experience working with physicians or supervising providers."**

**What they are really testing:** Collaboration style.

Because PA practice is fundamentally collaborative, organizations want clinicians who:

- respect the physician partnership model
- communicate clearly
- know when to escalate
- function confidently without ego conflict

Interviewers are assessing whether you can operate comfortably inside a team-based clinical structure.

**7. “What specialties interest you long term?”**

**What they are really testing:** Retention probability.

Employers understand that career interests evolve, but they want to see whether your interests align reasonably with the position they are hiring for. If you apply to emergency medicine but say your long-term goal is dermatology within six months, they may anticipate rapid turnover.

This question evaluates realistic alignment between role and candidate trajectory.

**8. “How do you manage stress?”**

**What they are really testing:** Sustainability.

Healthcare organizations are increasingly aware that burnout affects retention, patient care, and team morale. They want to understand:

- whether you recognize stress signals early
- whether you use healthy coping strategies
- whether you maintain functional performance under pressure

Strong answers demonstrate awareness and personal responsibility for resilience.

**9. “Tell us about a time you disagreed with a colleague.”**

**What they are really testing:** Professional conflict navigation.

Healthcare environments require constant collaboration

among strong personalities. Interviewers want clinicians who can:

- disagree respectfully
- communicate evidence-based reasoning
- prioritize patient care over ego
- preserve working relationships

This question evaluates maturity more than clinical knowledge.

**10. "Why do you want to work here?"**

**What they are really testing:** Preparation and intentionality.

Generic answers suggest low engagement. Hiring leaders want candidates who:

- researched the organization
- understand the department's patient population
- appreciate the culture or mission
- see themselves contributing meaningfully

Preparation signals professionalism and seriousness.

**Behavioral Question Patterns**

Many interviews now rely on **behavioral interviewing**, where candidates are asked to describe past experiences as predictors of future performance. These questions often begin with:

- "Tell me about a time when..."

- "Give an example of..."
- "Describe a situation where..."

The most effective way to answer is the **Situation → Action → Result** structure:

1 Briefly describe the situation

2 Explain the actions you took

3 Share the measurable or observable outcome

4 Add what you learned, when relevant

This structure demonstrates organized thinking and outcome awareness.

**Questions You Should Expect from Clinical Leadership**

Clinical directors often ask questions designed to evaluate operational readiness:

- "How comfortable are you managing uncertain diagnoses?"
- "How do you decide when to consult?"
- "What is your approach when patient expectations conflict with medical recommendations?"
- "How do you stay current with clinical guidelines?"

These questions are assessing judgment, humility, and learning orientation rather than memorized facts.

**What Interviewers Notice That Candidates Often Miss**

Even when answers are strong, interviewers are also observing:

- Communication clarity
- Listening skills
- Confidence without arrogance
- Ability to stay concise
- Professional demeanor with all staff members, not only interviewers
- Interaction with front desk or nursing staff during the visit

Hiring decisions are frequently influenced by how well candidates integrate socially and operationally into the team environment.

**Questions You Should Ask Them**

Intelligent interviews are two-directional. Asking thoughtful questions signals professionalism and helps you evaluate whether the position fits you as well.

Examples include:

- “How is productivity measured in this role?”
- “What qualities make someone successful in this department?”
- “How does the physician–PA collaboration typically function day to day?”
- “What support systems exist for new providers during the first year?”
- “What are the biggest challenges new PAs face here?”

These questions demonstrate maturity, long-term thinking, and alignment awareness.

**Final Perspective**

The purpose of an interview is not to prove perfection. It is to demonstrate **how you think, how you work, and how you respond when real-world complexity appears**. Hiring leaders are not searching for flawless candidates; they are searching for clinicians who can function safely, collaborate effectively, learn continuously, and sustain performance over time.

When you understand what interview questions are truly evaluating, the process becomes less about guessing the right answer and more about **accurately representing how you operate as a clinician** — which is ultimately what determines long-term success in Physician Assistant practice.

Chapter 52

# Behavioral Interviewing™ — Why It's Used, What It Measures, and How to Answer With Confidence

Behavioral interviewing has become the dominant interview style across healthcare systems because it is one of the most reliable ways to predict how someone will perform once hired. Clinical knowledge can be trained, workflows can be learned, and protocols can be memorized, but decision-making patterns, communication habits, emotional regulation, and professional accountability tend to remain consistent over time. Behavioral interviewing is designed to reveal those patterns.

Instead of asking hypothetical questions such as "What would you do if...," interviewers ask candidates to describe **what they have already done** in real situations. The assumption behind this approach is simple: past behavior is one of the strongest predictors of future behavior. When hiring leaders ask you to "tell me about a time," they are not testing your storytelling ability — they are evaluating how you think, how you respond under pressure, how you interact with colleagues, and how you take responsibility when outcomes are uncertain.

For Physician Assistants, behavioral interviewing is particularly important because the role sits at the intersection of clinical judgment, physician collaboration, patient communication, and operational efficiency. Hiring teams are not only assessing whether you can practice medicine safely; they are assessing whether you can function within the real pace and interpersonal complexity of their environment.

Most behavioral questions are designed to evaluate one of five areas: accountability, teamwork, communication, decision-making, or adaptability. Once you recognize this pattern, the questions become much easier to answer because you understand what the interviewer is truly looking for beneath the surface.

The most effective method for answering behavioral questions is the **Situation–Action–Result (SAR)** structure. First, briefly describe the situation so the listener understands the context. Second, explain the specific actions you took — not what the team did, but what you personally contributed. Third, describe the result and what changed because of your actions. When appropriate, include what you learned from the experience. This structured approach demonstrates organized thinking, accountability, and outcome awareness, all of which signal professional maturity.

Below are common behavioral interview themes for Physician Assistants, along with example response frameworks that illustrate how to answer confidently and professionally.

### Handling a Difficult Patient Interaction

Interviewers frequently ask: "Tell me about a time you handled a difficult patient or family interaction."

What they are evaluating is emotional regulation, communication skill, and professionalism under stress.

**Script Framework:**

"In one of my clinical rotations, I worked with a patient who was frustrated because their treatment plan was not improving symptoms as quickly as expected. The situation became tense, and I recognized that the patient felt unheard. I took time to listen without interrupting, acknowledged the frustration, and clarified the treatment goals in plain language. I then reviewed the care plan with the supervising provider to ensure consistency in messaging. After the discussion, the patient expressed a better understanding of the plan and agreed to continue the recommended treatment. That experience reinforced for me how much de-escalation and patient trust depend on clear communication and empathy."

This response shows listening, composure, collaboration, and resolution — the real traits being measured.

**Working Through a Clinical Uncertainty**

Another common question: "Tell me about a time you were unsure of a clinical decision."

This evaluates judgment, humility, and patient-safety awareness.

**Script Framework:**

"During a rotation, I evaluated a patient whose symptoms suggested multiple possible diagnoses. I completed the initial assessment and developed a preliminary differential, but I recognized that additional evaluation was needed before finalizing a plan. I discussed the case with the supervising physician, presented my reasoning, and asked targeted questions about next steps. Together we refined the diagnostic approach and ordered additional tests. The final diagnosis differed slightly from my initial thinking, and the case strengthened my understanding of how collaborative consultation improves accuracy and patient safety."

This demonstrates sound reasoning and willingness to seek guidance — qualities hiring teams value highly.

**Managing a Heavy Workload**

Interviewers often ask: "Describe a time you had to manage competing priorities."

This measures workflow organization, prioritization, and resilience.

**Script Framework:**

"During a high-volume clinic day, I was responsible for assisting with multiple patient evaluations while also completing documentation responsibilities. I prioritized patients based on acuity and urgency, communicated clearly with the nursing staff about workflow adjustments, and documented in short intervals throughout the day rather than waiting until the end. By the end of the shift, all patients had been evaluated safely, and documentation remained current. That experience reinforced my approach of prioritizing patient safety first while maintaining steady documentation habits to prevent backlog."

This shows operational thinking and sustainability under pressure.

**Resolving a Team Conflict**

Another behavioral prompt may be: "Tell me about a time you disagreed with a colleague."

This evaluates professionalism, conflict navigation, and team maturity.

**Script Framework:**

"In one clinical setting, a colleague and I initially disagreed about the urgency of a patient follow-up. Rather than debating the issue informally, we reviewed the patient's chart together and discussed the clinical reasoning behind each perspective. After clarifying the patient's risk factors, we aligned on a plan that prioritized earlier follow-up. The experience reminded me that disagreements are often opportunities to improve decision quality when they are handled respectfully and focused on patient outcomes."

Hiring leaders listen for respectful collaboration rather than dominance or avoidance.

**Adapting to Change**

Healthcare environments change rapidly, so interviewers frequently ask: "Tell me about a time you had to adapt quickly."

This assesses flexibility and learning speed.

**Script Framework:**

"During a clinical rotation, workflow changes were introduced that required a different documentation process and patient routing system. Initially, the adjustment slowed the team, but I spent time learning the updated process, asked experienced staff for tips, and created a quick-reference checklist for myself to stay organized. Within a short time, I was able to maintain efficiency again, and the experience reinforced the importance of adaptability in fast-changing clinical environments."

This demonstrates resilience and proactive learning.

**Why Behavioral Interviewing Matters for Long-Term Fit**

Behavioral interviewing is not designed to intimidate candidates; it is designed to reduce hiring risk. Healthcare organizations invest significant time and resources onboarding new clinicians, and turnover can destabilize teams quickly. By understanding how candidates have behaved in real situations — how they respond to uncertainty, stress, teamwork challenges, and responsibility — hiring leaders gain a clearer picture of whether someone will thrive in their environment.

For candidates, understanding behavioral interviewing transforms the experience from stressful guesswork into structured storytelling. Instead of trying to invent perfect answers, you draw from real experiences that demonstrate professionalism, decision-making, and growth. Preparing several strong examples in advance — one involving teamwork, one involving challenge, one involving learning, and one involving patient communication — ensures you are ready for most behavioral questions you will encounter.

**Preparation Strategy**

Before interviews, identify five real experiences from clinical rotations, early practice, volunteer work, or employment that demonstrate responsibility, learning, collaboration, and resilience. Write brief notes using the Situation–Action–Result structure and practice explaining them clearly in under two minutes. Preparation does not make your answers sound scripted; it makes them organized and confident.

**Final Perspective**

Behavioral interviewing exists because technical knowledge alone does not determine success in healthcare roles. Sustainability, teamwork, emotional steadiness, communication clarity, and decision discipline shape daily performance far more than memorized facts. When you answer behavioral questions with structured, honest examples, you allow hiring teams to see how you truly operate — and that clarity benefits both sides of the hiring decision.

Chapter 53

# Terms of Care™

Negotiation in healthcare is rarely taught and almost never modeled well. Most PAs learn by inference, awkward conversations, or post-hoc regret. Terms of Care™ exists to change that by reframing negotiation as professional alignment rather than personal advocacy.

This is not about "getting more." It is about understanding what you are actually agreeing to when you say yes—and whether that agreement is sustainable over time.

Every offer contains explicit terms and implicit expectations. Salary is only the visible surface. The real agreement lives underneath it, in workload, availability, support, boundaries, and exit conditions. Terms of Care™ teaches you to read both layers before they cost you something you didn't intend to trade.

***Total Compensation Is Not Salary***

Most PAs fixate on base pay because it is easy to compare and emotionally salient. Employers know this. That is why many offers look competitive on paper while shifting cost elsewhere.

Total compensation includes salary, benefits, schedule, call burden, productivity expectations, documentation time, CME support, licensure coverage, malpractice structure, and long-term flexibility. A slightly lower salary paired with protected time, strong onboarding, and predictable scheduling often outperforms a higher salary in real life.

The critical skill is learning to model tradeoffs honestly. Ask yourself what the offer requires weekly, monthly, and annually —not just financially, but cognitively and emotionally. If the numbers look good but the structure feels brittle, that is not generosity. It is leverage.

### *Call, Coverage, and the Quiet Expansion of Scope*

Call expectations are one of the most common sources of misalignment, especially when described casually. "Shared call," "light call," or "rotating call" are not terms of precision. They are placeholders for future negotiation—or future frustration.

Clarify frequency, duration, backup, and compensation. Ask how call has changed in the last year. Ask what happens when someone leaves. Ask who absorbs coverage gaps. These questions are not confrontational; they are predictive.

A role that relies on goodwill to sustain coverage is unstable by design.

### *Productivity, Metrics, and Moving Targets*

Productivity expectations are rarely fixed, even when numbers are provided. RVUs, patient volume, and panel size often drift upward as systems adjust to staffing pressure. The question is not whether productivity is measured—it almost always is—but whether it is contextualized.

Ask how metrics are used. Are they informational or punitive? Are they adjusted for acuity, staffing, or complexity? Are they tied to compensation without clear guardrails?

When expectations are vague, pressure fills the gap.

### *Documentation Time Is Work Time*

One of the most common hidden costs in PA roles is uncompensated documentation. When charting is expected to spill into evenings or days off, the role is quietly extracting time without naming it.

Ask how documentation time is accounted for. Ask whether notes are expected to be completed during scheduled hours. Ask how often clinicians chart at home. These questions surface cultural norms that contracts rarely capture.

If documentation expectations are unrealistic, no amount of efficiency will fix the imbalance.

### *CME, Licensure, and Professional Maintenance*

CME funds, licensure fees, DEA coverage, and professional memberships are not perks. They are maintenance costs of practicing safely and legally. When these are underfunded or conditional, the burden shifts to you.

Clarify not just the dollar amount, but the ease of use. Funds that exist but are difficult to access may as well not exist. The same applies to time off for education. Financial support without time is incomplete.

Professional growth requires more than permission. It requires structure.

### *Noncompetes and Exit Language*

Exit terms matter most when things don't go as planned—which is precisely when you have the least leverage. Noncompete clauses, notice periods, and repayment obligations can constrain future options in ways that are difficult to unwind.

Read these sections slowly. Ask how often they are enforced. Ask what happens if the role changes materially. Ask how departures have been handled historically. These questions do not signal disloyalty. They signal foresight.

A good role should not trap you to retain you.

### *How to Negotiate Without Burning Capital*

Effective negotiation is calm and specific. It is not adversarial. The strongest approach is collaborative clarification: naming what you need to succeed and asking whether the role can support that.

Avoid ultimatums. Avoid emotional framing. Use structure instead. "In order to be effective long term, I need..." is stronger than "I was hoping for..." The former frames negotiation as alignment. The latter frames it as preference.

Silence after a counteroffer is normal. Give it space. Confidence reads quieter than urgency.

### *When to Walk Away*

The hardest skill in negotiation is knowing when the answer is no—not because the offer is bad, but because the misalignment is structural. If key concerns are minimized, deflected, or left vague, assume they will not improve after hire.

Walking away early is not failure. It is preservation. The cost of a misaligned role compounds faster than the cost of waiting for a better fit.

### *The Terms of Care™ Rule to Lock*

If you cannot explain the full agreement to yourself clearly—what you give, what you get, and what happens if things change—you do not yet understand the offer well enough to accept it.

Negotiation is not about winning. It is about entering a role with eyes open and boundaries intact.

That is alignment in practice.

Chapter 54

# Terms of Care™ — Negotiation Scripts That Don't Cost You Trust

Most PAs don't avoid negotiation because they lack leverage. They avoid it because they don't want to damage relationships before they start. That instinct is understandable—and exploitable. Employers expect questions. What they react poorly to is emotional framing, vagueness, or ultimatums.

Effective negotiation language is calm, specific, and future-oriented. It frames requests as requirements for effectiveness rather than personal desires. The difference matters.

Instead of saying, "I was hoping for a higher salary," anchor the conversation in function: *"To be effective and sustainable in this role, I need clarity around workload expectations and how compensation reflects them."* This signals professionalism, not entitlement.

When addressing salary directly, specificity beats defensiveness. *"Based on the scope, call expectations, and market data for this role, I was expecting something closer to*

*X. Is there flexibility there?"* This opens a conversation without forcing confrontation.

If the answer is no, listen to what replaces it. Strong offers rarely say no without offering alternatives. Weak offers deflect or minimize.

***Call and Coverage — Scripts That Surface Reality***

Call is one of the most common sources of long-term misalignment because it expands quietly. The right questions are not accusatory; they are predictive.

Useful phrasing sounds like this: *"Can you walk me through how call is handled when someone is out or leaves the team?"* or *"How has call changed over the last year?"* These questions force reflection without blame.

If answers are vague or overly optimistic, assume instability. Precision in answers usually reflects experience managing the issue. Evasion suggests reliance on goodwill rather than structure.

***Productivity Expectations — Clarifying Moving Targets***

When productivity is discussed, many offers include numbers without context. Your job is to supply the missing structure.

Ask how productivity is measured and used. *"Are these metrics primarily informational, or are they tied to compensation or performance review?"* Follow with, *"How are they adjusted when staffing or acuity changes?"*

If adjustments are informal or discretionary, that discretion will eventually be exercised—often under pressure. Clarity protects both sides.

### ***Documentation Time — Naming the Invisible Labor***

Documentation expectations are rarely stated outright, yet they shape quality of life profoundly. The script here should be neutral and practical: *"What is the expectation around completing documentation during scheduled hours versus after hours?"* Follow with, *"How common is charting from home in this role?"*

These questions normalize the issue rather than framing it as a complaint. If the answer is "everyone charts at home sometimes," ask how often and for how long. Vague reassurance is not a plan.

### ***CME and Professional Maintenance — Separating Permission from Support***

When CME is mentioned, clarify both funding and time. *"Is CME time protected, or does it come from PTO?"* and *"How easy is it to access CME funds in practice?"* These questions often reveal whether professional growth is encouraged or merely allowed.

Support that exists on paper but is difficult to use is not real support.

### ***Noncompetes and Exit Terms — Asking Without Alarm***

Many PAs hesitate to ask about noncompetes or exit clauses because they fear signaling disloyalty. In reality, mature organizations expect these questions.

A simple script works: *"Can you help me understand how this noncompete has been applied in the past?"* or *"What happens if the role changes materially after hire?"* These questions frame exit terms as contingencies, not intentions.

If answers are defensive, take note. Healthy systems don't rely on fear to retain people.

### ***Red-Flag Language to Decode***

Certain phrases appear benign but often signal future strain.

"Fast-paced" without staffing ratios usually means chronic overload.

"Flexible" without boundaries often means unpredictable.

"We're like a family" can mean blurred lines around availability.

"You'll grow into it" sometimes means the role is not yet well-defined.

None of these automatically disqualify a role, but all of them demand follow-up.

### ***When Negotiation Reveals the Answer***

Sometimes negotiation doesn't improve an offer—it clarifies it. If key questions are minimized, deferred, or reframed as attitude issues, the misalignment is already present. No amount of goodwill will resolve structural ambiguity.

Walking away in those moments is not premature. It is disciplined.

### ***The Terms of Care™ Decision Test (Lock This)***

Before accepting any offer, you should be able to answer three questions without hesitation:

What am I being paid for—explicitly and implicitly?

What support structures make this sustainable?

What happens if circumstances change?

If any of those answers are unclear, the negotiation is not finished—or the role is not aligned.

Chapter 55

# Next Steps — Practicing With Intention

If you are stepping into your first PA role, the most important next step is not mastery. It is stabilization. Focus on building reliable habits before expanding scope. Learn how your system actually functions rather than how it is described. Identify who answers questions well, who cuts corners, and where risk quietly accumulates. Early competence is not about speed; it is about consistency and judgment.

As your footing strengthens, revisit the systems in this book deliberately. Resume language should evolve as responsibility grows. Interview strategies should sharpen as your leverage increases. Negotiation should become calmer, not more aggressive. Alignment is easier to protect when you treat each transition as a decision rather than an inevitability.

For those further along, the next step may be refinement rather than change. Adjusting setting, schedule, or scope can restore sustainability without abandoning the profession. Small structural shifts often matter more than dramatic exits.

The question to keep asking is not "What else could I do?" but "What version of this work fits who I am now?"

### *Professional Anchors and Communities*

No PA practices in isolation, even when it feels that way. Professional communities matter—not as résumé lines, but as anchors. Associations, specialty groups, and peer networks provide perspective that individual workplaces cannot. They remind you that your experience is contextual, not personal.

Engage selectively. Look for spaces that encourage honest discussion rather than constant optimization. Pay attention to how leaders talk about boundaries, workload, and longevity. Culture travels through language long before it shows up in policy.

Mentorship is especially valuable when it is informal and reciprocal. Seek out clinicians who practice in ways you respect, not just those with impressive titles. The most useful mentors are often the ones who can articulate what they stopped tolerating and why.

### *Learning That Lasts*

Continuing education should not be treated as maintenance alone. Over time, it becomes a way to shape your career deliberately. Choose learning that aligns with the direction you are moving, not just the requirements you must meet. Depth often matters more than breadth.

Be cautious of equating constant upskilling with progress. Learning that adds responsibility without support can increase strain rather than satisfaction. The goal is not to accumulate credentials, but to build a practice that remains coherent as complexity increases.

### *A Note on Staying Present*

Healthcare rewards vigilance. It rarely rewards presence. The difference matters.

Staying present means noticing when your work begins to crowd out recovery. It means recognizing when pride turns into pressure. It means allowing yourself to pause before momentum hardens into obligation. None of this requires dramatic action. It requires attention.

Careers drift when reflection is postponed indefinitely.

### *Acknowledgments*

This book exists because countless Physician Assistants were willing to speak honestly about their work—the parts that inspire them and the parts that quietly cost more than expected. Their experiences shaped the questions this book asks and the systems it offers in response.

It also exists because readers were willing to slow down long enough to consider fit before committing fully. That choice alone places you ahead of most.

Finally, this work reflects a belief that healthcare careers deserve more than generic advice. They deserve language that respects complexity, systems that protect sustainability, and frameworks that treat alignment as essential rather than optional.

### *Closing*

You will not outgrow the need for alignment. You will outgrow roles that no longer fit. That is not failure. It is movement.

Return to these questions when decisions feel rushed. Revisit these systems when opportunities feel flattering but unclear. Trust that clarity often arrives quietly, and that listening early costs less than repairing later.

The work continues.

So does your ability to choose it well.

## Chapter 56
# The Never End

***The Never End — Physician Assistant Edition***

If you've made it this far, something important has already happened. You didn't just learn about the Physician Assistant role. You tested it—against your values, your tolerance, your identity, and your future self. That matters more than enthusiasm ever will.

Most career books end with reassurance. This one ends with responsibility.

Not responsibility in the sense of obligation to a system or a title, but responsibility to yourself. To notice when fit holds. To act when it doesn't. To understand that careers in healthcare are not linear journeys toward certainty, but ongoing negotiations between who you are and what the work requires of you.

That negotiation never really ends.

***Choosing the PA Role—Again and Again***

Becoming a Physician Assistant is not a one-time decision. It is a choice you make repeatedly—when you select a setting, when you negotiate boundaries, when you accept or decline added responsibility, when you decide whether to stay or pivot. The title stays the same. The lived experience does not.

Early in a PA career, momentum does much of the choosing for you. Training funnels you forward. Opportunities appear quickly. Saying yes feels easier than slowing down to ask whether the structure supports you long term. That's normal. It's also temporary.

As your competence grows, so does your agency. The danger is assuming that agency will automatically be offered. It rarely is. It must be claimed intentionally, using the same discernment you applied when choosing the profession in the first place.

Alignment is not something you "find" and keep forever. It is something you reassess as responsibilities shift, life expands, and systems change around you.

### *There Is No Perfect Role—Only Honest Tradeoffs*

Every PA role comes with tradeoffs. Some are obvious. Others reveal themselves slowly. The mistake is not choosing a role with compromises. The mistake is pretending compromises don't exist until they accumulate into resentment or exhaustion.

You are allowed to want meaningful work *and* a life that fits outside of it. You are allowed to value competence without sacrificing health. You are allowed to redefine success as your priorities change.

Healthcare culture often frames these adjustments as weakness. They are not. They are evidence of maturity.

The strongest PAs are not the ones who endure the most. They are the ones who adapt early enough to preserve themselves.

### ***Professional Growth Without Disappearance***

One of the quiet risks in healthcare careers is identity collapse—when your role absorbs more of you than you intended. Titles become shorthand for worth. Productivity becomes proxy for value. Over time, everything else narrows.

Resist that.

Being a PA is meaningful work. It should not be the only place where meaning is allowed to live. Careers that crowd out everything else eventually feel heavier than they should.

Sustainability requires expansion, not contraction. Interests outside of medicine. Relationships not defined by schedules. Space to be human without performing usefulness.

You do not owe the profession your whole identity.

### ***Staying Versus Leaving***

At some point, most PAs confront a difficult question: *Is this still right for me?* The answer may be yes, with adjustment. It may be no, without regret. What matters is not the direction you choose, but whether you choose deliberately.

Leaving a role—or even the profession—does not invalidate what you gave to it. Staying does not obligate you to tolerate harm. Both paths require honesty.

If you stay, stay with boundaries. If you pivot, pivot without shame.

Misalignment ignored tends to announce itself later, more loudly, and at a higher cost.

### *Your Responsibility Going Forward*

You now understand the systems. Hiring. Interviewing. Negotiation. Onboarding. The tolls that appear quietly. The signals that matter. That knowledge creates responsibility—not to do everything perfectly, but to notice when something feels off and respond before damage accumulates.

Pay attention to how your body responds to work. Pay attention to what drains you disproportionately. Pay attention to what restores you. These are not side effects. They are data.

Revisit alignment regularly. Especially when opportunities arise quickly. Especially when praise increases. Especially when exhaustion is framed as normal.

The cost of ignoring misalignment is rarely immediate. That is why it is so dangerous.

### *Where This Book Connects Forward*

This book was designed to help you *decide*, not to tell you what to choose. If you want a broader view—across hundreds of healthcare roles, future paths, and alignment patterns—*What Color Are Your Scrubs?* expands this framework beyond the PA profession. It exists to help you zoom out when you need to, without losing yourself in options.

If you want a more personalized mirror, the **SCRUB*fit*™ Healthcare Career Assessment** was built to capture patterns over time, not snapshots. It prioritizes sustainability over capability and fit over fantasy. Used thoughtfully, it becomes a checkpoint you can return to as your career evolves.

Neither tool replaces judgment. Both support it.

***The Never End***

Healthcare careers don't end with answers. They continue through better questions.

If you are honest with yourself, you will change. If you are attentive, your career can change with you instead of against you. If you are willing to pause before momentum hardens into habit, you can design a path that remains viable—not just impressive.

That is the work most people postpone.

You didn't.

So don't rush the next step. Don't outsource decisions to expectation. Don't assume endurance is the same as alignment.

This is not the end of the journey.

It is the point where you know how to keep choosing well.

Goodbye for now,

ScrubTales™ Physician Assistant

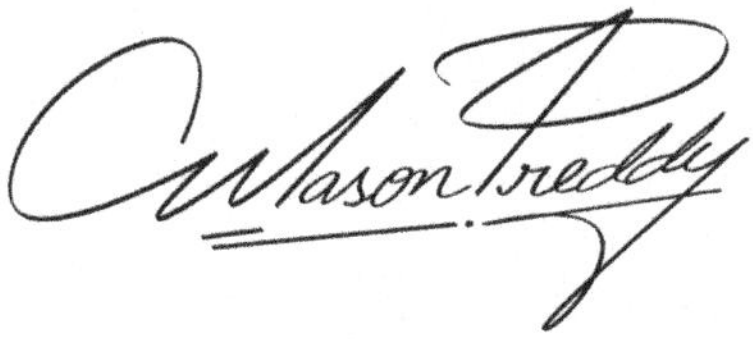

Chapter 57

# Glossary

**Glossary — 100 Terms Every Physician Assistant Should Begin Learning**

Healthcare has its own language, and much of it is absorbed informally—through observation, repetition, and quiet correction—rather than taught outright. For Physician Assistants, this can create an uneven learning curve. You may recognize terms long before you truly understand how they shape workload, risk, identity, and sustainability in practice.

This glossary exists to level that field.

The terms included here are not random vocabulary. They are concepts you will encounter repeatedly as a PA—during training, hiring, onboarding, negotiation, and long-term practice. Some describe clinical realities. Others describe systems, structures, and pressures that influence how the work actually feels. Together, they form a shared language for noticing alignment, naming strain, and making informed decisions over time.

You are not expected to master these terms immediately. You are expected to begin recognizing them. Fluency develops through use, reflection, and experience. This glossary gives you a place to return when something feels familiar but unsettled—when you need language to clarify what you're experiencing rather than normalize it away.

**A**

**Accountability**

The responsibility to answer for clinical decisions and outcomes, regardless of how much authority accompanies the role. For PAs, accountability often exists even when control over staffing, workflow, or policy does not, creating tension if not acknowledged.

**Acuity**

The severity and complexity of patient conditions that determine pace, risk, and cognitive demand. Acuity influences workload far more than raw patient volume and is frequently underestimated in role descriptions.

**Alignment**

The degree to which a role fits how you are wired, how you carry responsibility, and what you need to remain sustainable over time. Alignment is not enthusiasm or competence; it is compatibility between identity and structure.

**Autonomy**

The ability to make independent clinical decisions within a role. Autonomy is shaped by supervision agreements, institutional culture, and trust, and it expands or contracts depending on context.

## B

### Boundary Setting

The professional skill of defining limits around time, scope, availability, and responsibility. Effective boundaries protect patient safety and clinician sustainability rather than undermining commitment.

### Burnout

A state of emotional exhaustion, detachment, and reduced sense of efficacy that often reflects prolonged misalignment rather than personal failure. Burnout is frequently treated as an individual issue despite being structurally produced.

## C

### Call

Any obligation to be available outside scheduled clinical hours. Call expectations vary widely and are a common source of hidden workload expansion when poorly defined.

### Capacity

The realistic amount of clinical, cognitive, and emotional work that can be carried safely at a given time. Capacity fluctuates with acuity, staffing, and life circumstances, yet is often treated as fixed.

### Clinical Judgment

The ability to synthesize information, assess risk, and make decisions under uncertainty. Clinical judgment develops over time and cannot be reduced to protocols alone.

**Clinical Load**

The combined burden of patient volume, acuity, documentation, coordination, and follow-up required in a role. Clinical load is more predictive of fatigue than patient count alone.

**Cognitive Load**

The total mental effort required to perform work, including vigilance, multitasking, and decision-making. Sustained high cognitive load without recovery increases error risk and exhaustion.

## D

**Decision Fatigue**

The depletion of mental resources caused by repeated decision-making without adequate recovery. Decision fatigue reduces judgment quality and increases emotional strain.

**Documentation Burden**

The time and cognitive cost associated with clinical documentation, particularly when charting extends beyond scheduled hours. Documentation burden is a major driver of dissatisfaction.

## E

**Emotional Labor**

The effort required to regulate emotions, manage interpersonal dynamics, and maintain professionalism under stress. Emotional labor is real work that is rarely acknowledged explicitly.

**Escalation**

The act of involving additional expertise or authority when uncertainty, risk, or scope boundaries require it. Appropriate escalation reflects professionalism, not inadequacy.

**Expectation Drift**

The gradual expansion of responsibilities beyond what was originally agreed upon, often without formal discussion. Expectation drift is a common precursor to burnout.

**F**

**Fit**

The practical expression of alignment within a specific role, setting, and team. Fit is contextual and can change over time even when skills remain strong.

**G**

**Growth Path**

The trajectory through which responsibility, scope, and expectations evolve over time. Healthy growth paths are intentional rather than assumed.

**H**

**Hidden Labor**

Work that is expected but not formally recognized or compensated, such as after-hours charting, informal coverage, or emotional regulation. Hidden labor accumulates quietly.

## I

### Institutional Memory

Knowledge of how an organization actually functions beyond written policy. While useful, institutional memory can normalize dysfunction if left unexamined.

### Intelligent Interviews

A hiring approach that focuses on decoding risk, expectations, and structure rather than performing enthusiasm. Intelligent interviews prioritize clarity over impressing.

## J

### Judgment Under Pressure

The ability to make sound decisions in high-stakes, time-constrained situations. This skill depends heavily on support structures, not just experience.

## L

### Leverage

The ability to influence terms, expectations, or decisions. Leverage changes over time and is shaped by experience, scarcity, and specialization.

### Liability Exposure

The degree of legal and professional risk associated with a role. Liability exposure is influenced by supervision, documentation practices, and institutional support.

## M

### Moral Distress

Psychological discomfort that arises when clinicians know the ethically appropriate action but are constrained from taking it. Moral distress is a structural signal, not a personal flaw.

**N**

**Normalization of Deviance**

The gradual acceptance of unsafe or unsustainable practices as normal because they are common. This process erodes standards over time.

**O**

**Onboarding**

The structured period during which a new hire is supported, supervised, and integrated into a role. Effective onboarding reduces risk and accelerates confidence.

**On-Call Creep**

The slow expansion of call responsibilities beyond original agreements, often framed as temporary but rarely reversed without renegotiation.

**P**

**Panel Interview**

An interview format involving multiple stakeholders that often reveals cultural dynamics more clearly than one-on-one conversations.

**Performance Metrics**

Quantitative measures used to assess output or quality. Metrics become harmful when divorced from context.

**Psychological Safety**

The sense that one can ask questions, admit uncertainty, or raise concerns without fear of punishment. Psychological safety is foundational to learning.

**R**

**Red Flag**

A signal—often subtle—that suggests misalignment, instability, or risk. Red flags are predictive patterns, not isolated incidents.

**Role Creep**

The expansion of responsibilities without corresponding authority, compensation, or support. Role creep is a leading driver of PA dissatisfaction.

**S**

**Scope of Practice**

The activities a PA is legally and institutionally permitted to perform. Scope is shaped as much by culture as by regulation.

**SCRUBScript™**

A structured approach to resume development that evolves with experience and responsibility rather than remaining static.

**Supervision**

The formal and informal systems that support clinical decision-making. Effective supervision evolves over time.

**Sustainability**

The ability to perform a role over time without disproportionate cost to health, identity, or relationships.

**T**

**Team Load Distribution**

How work and responsibility are divided across a clinical team. Uneven distribution drives resentment and burnout.

**Terms of Care™**

The framework used to evaluate compensation, workload, expectations, and boundaries in healthcare job offers.

**Total Compensation**

The full value of an offer, including salary, benefits, schedule, call burden, and support—not just base pay.

**Turnover Signal**

Patterns such as frequent job reposting or leadership churn that indicate systemic strain.

**U**

**Uncertainty Tolerance**

The ability to function effectively when information is incomplete. This capacity is shaped by support structures as much as experience.

**Unpaid Time**

Work performed outside compensated hours, often normalized through culture rather than policy.

**W**

**Workflow Friction**

Inefficiencies in systems or processes that increase cognitive load and slow care delivery.

**Workflow Ownership**

Responsibility for managing patient flow and coordination, often assigned without authority or support.

**Z**

**Zone of Sustainability**

The range in which workload, responsibility, and recovery remain balanced enough to support long-term practice.

Chapter 58

# 100 More BONUS Glossary Entries

Healthcare is a language of precision, speed, and shared understanding. In clinical environments, communication does not slow down to explain terminology, abbreviations, or procedural language; it moves quickly, and those who understand the vocabulary can participate confidently in patient care conversations, documentation, and clinical decision-making. For Physician Assistants, developing familiarity with commonly used clinical terms is not about memorization for its own sake — it is about reducing hesitation, improving clarity, and functioning more effectively within interdisciplinary teams.

The following glossary is designed as a practical learning bridge. These are not obscure academic terms, but the types of words, phrases, and shorthand that appear repeatedly in charting, handoffs, consults, patient discussions, and team communication. Becoming comfortable with this vocabulary early allows new and future PAs to focus less on decoding language and more on understanding patient context, clinical reasoning, and workflow priorities.

You are not expected to master every term immediately. Instead, treat this section as an ongoing reference. Revisit it as you encounter unfamiliar language in clinical rotations, early practice experiences, or interdisciplinary discussions. Over time, what once required translation becomes second nature — and fluency in the language of healthcare becomes one more factor that strengthens confidence, efficiency, and professional presence in the Physician Assistant role.

**The 100 More Words Every Physician Assistant Should Begin Learning**

Below are 100 commonly encountered clinical terms Physician Assistants will hear in documentation, rounds, handoffs, and interdisciplinary discussions. These are working-language terms intended to build early fluency in clinical communication.

**1. Acuity**

The severity of a patient's condition and the level of care required.

**2. Adherence**

The degree to which a patient follows a prescribed treatment plan.

**3. Adverse Event**

An unintended injury or complication caused by healthcare management rather than the disease itself.

**4. Algorithm**

A structured clinical decision pathway used to guide diagnosis or treatment.

**5. Ambulate**

To walk or assist a patient in walking.

**6. Analgesia**

Pain relief or the absence of pain sensation.

**7. Anamnesis**

A patient's medical history obtained during clinical questioning.

**8. Anticoagulation**

Medication therapy used to reduce blood clot formation.

**9. Assessment**

The clinician's evaluation and interpretation of patient findings.

**10. Asymptomatic**

Presenting without symptoms.

**11. Baseline**

A patient's normal or usual health status used for comparison.

**12. Biopsy**

Removal of tissue for diagnostic examination.

**13. Breakthrough Pain**

Pain that occurs despite ongoing pain-control therapy.

**14. Care Coordination**

Organization of patient care activities across providers and settings.

**15. Case Presentation**

A structured verbal summary of a patient's condition and plan.

**16. Chief Complaint**

The primary reason a patient seeks care.

**17. Chronic**

A condition lasting longer than three months or ongoing.

**18. Clinical Judgment**

Decision-making based on knowledge, experience, and patient context.

**19. Comorbidity**

The presence of additional diseases occurring with a primary condition.

**20. Compliance**

Patient cooperation with treatment recommendations.

**21. Consult**

Request for specialist evaluation or guidance.

**22. Contraindication**

A factor that makes a treatment inadvisable.

**23. Critical Value**

A laboratory result indicating immediate clinical concern.

**24. Differential Diagnosis**

A list of possible conditions explaining a patient's symptoms.

**25. Discharge Planning**

Preparation for patient transition from a healthcare facility.

**26. Documentation Burden**

The workload associated with clinical charting requirements.

**27. Downtime**

Periods when clinical systems, especially electronic records, are unavailable.

**28. Early Intervention**

Treatment started at an early stage to improve outcomes.

**29. Escalation of Care**

Increasing the level of medical support when a patient worsens.

**30. Evidence-Based Practice**

Clinical decisions guided by research, expertise, and patient values.

**31. Exacerbation**

A worsening of a disease or symptoms.

**32. Follow-Up**

Subsequent evaluation after treatment or initial visit.

**33. Formulary**

A list of medications approved for use within a healthcare system.

**34. Functional Status**

A patient's ability to perform daily activities.

**35. Guideline**

A systematically developed recommendation for clinical practice.

**36. Hand-Off**

Transfer of patient responsibility between clinicians.

**37. Hemodynamic Stability**

Stable blood circulation and vital signs.

**38. High-Risk Patient**

A patient with increased likelihood of complications.

**39. HPI (History of Present Illness)**

Detailed account of the development of the patient's current symptoms.

**40. Iatrogenic**

A condition caused by medical treatment.

**41. Informed Consent**

Patient authorization after understanding risks and benefits.

**42. Inpatient**

A patient admitted to the hospital.

**43. Interdisciplinary Team**

Healthcare professionals from multiple specialties working together.

**44. Intervention**

A medical action taken to treat or prevent disease.

**45. Length of Stay (LOS)**

The duration of a hospital admission.

**46. Level of Care**

The intensity of services required by a patient.

**47. Longitudinal Care**

Continuous healthcare management over time.

**48. Morbidity**

The presence of illness or disease.

**49. Mortality**

Death rate within a population.

**50. Multimodal Therapy**

Treatment using multiple methods simultaneously.

**51. Negative Predictive Value**

Likelihood that a negative test truly indicates absence of disease.

**52. Noncompliance**

Failure to follow prescribed treatment recommendations.

**53. Observation Status**

Hospital monitoring without full admission.

**54. Onset**

The beginning of symptoms.

**55. Outpatient**

A patient treated without hospital admission.

**56. Palliative Care**

Care focused on symptom relief and quality of life.

**57. Pathophysiology**

Functional changes associated with disease.

**58. Patient Throughput**

The rate at which patients move through a healthcare setting.

**59. Pharmacotherapy**

Treatment using medications.

**60. Polypharmacy**

Use of multiple medications simultaneously.

**61. Positive Predictive Value**

Likelihood that a positive test truly indicates disease.

**62. Post-Operative**

After a surgical procedure.

**63. Pre-Operative**

Before a surgical procedure.

**64. Preventive Care**

Services intended to prevent disease.

**65. Prognosis**

Expected outcome of a disease.

**66. Protocol**

A standardized clinical procedure or treatment plan.

**67. Provider**

A licensed healthcare professional delivering care.

**68. Quality Improvement (QI)**

Efforts to enhance patient care outcomes and processes.

**69. Readmission**

Return to the hospital after discharge.

**70. Referral**

Directing a patient to another provider for care.

**71. Regimen**

A structured treatment plan.

**72. Remission**

Reduction or disappearance of disease signs.

**73. Risk Stratification**

Categorizing patients by likelihood of adverse outcomes.

**74. Screening**

Testing asymptomatic individuals for disease detection.

**75. Sequelae**

Conditions resulting from a previous disease.

**76. Shared Decision-Making**

Clinician and patient collaborating on care decisions.

**77. Specialty Care**

Healthcare focused on a specific field of medicine.

**78. Stabilization**

Bringing a patient's condition under control.

**79. Standard of Care**

Accepted level of treatment provided by professionals.

**80. Symptomatic**

Showing symptoms of disease.

**81. Triage**

Prioritizing patients based on urgency.

**82. Turnaround Time**

Time required to receive test results or complete services.

**83. Utilization Review**

Evaluation of healthcare services for necessity and efficiency.

**84. Vital Signs**

Core physiologic measurements such as blood pressure and heart rate.

**85. Volume Status**

Assessment of fluid levels within the body.

**86. Workup**

Diagnostic evaluation process.

**87. Workflow Efficiency**

Optimization of clinical processes to improve care delivery.

**88. Worsening Trend**

Progressive deterioration in patient indicators.

**89. Acute**

A sudden onset condition with short duration.

**90. Benign**

Not harmful or cancerous.

**91. Chronic Management**

Ongoing care for long-term conditions.

**92. Clinical Course**

The progression of a disease over time.

**93. Debridement**

Removal of damaged tissue to aid healing.

**94. Diagnostic Yield**

Effectiveness of a test in identifying disease.

**95. Empiric Treatment**

Treatment started before a definitive diagnosis.

**96. Etiology**

Cause of a disease.

**97. Exclusion Criteria**

Conditions that prevent participation in a treatment or study.

**98. Indication**

A valid reason to use a specific treatment.

**99. Reconciliation (Medication)**

Verification of patient medication lists for accuracy.

**100. Therapeutic Response**

The patient's reaction to a treatment intervention.

# About the Author

Mason Preddy is a healthcare workforce strategist, recruiter, and publishing founder with more than **two and a half decades of experience in healthcare recruitment, retention, and workforce strategy**. Over the course of his career, he has worked closely with hospitals, health systems, academic medical centers, physician groups, and healthcare leaders across the United States, helping organizations understand not only how to hire clinicians — but how to retain them, support them, and align them with roles where they can sustainably thrive.

Throughout thousands of recruitment conversations, Mason observed a consistent pattern: most healthcare professionals did not leave the field because they lacked skill, intelligence, or compassion. They left because they found themselves working in environments, specialties, or role structures that did not align with how they were wired to function. This realization became the foundation for his long-standing focus on **career alignment**, identity-based role selection, and long-term workforce sustainability.

As the founder of Mason Maison™ Publishing, Mason created the **ScrubTales™** series and the broader **SCRUB*fit*™** career-alignment ecosystem to help future and current healthcare professionals understand the lived reality of clinical careers before committing years of education, financial investment, and emotional energy. His work emphasizes that choosing a healthcare career is not simply an academic decision or a salary calculation; it is a long-term identity decision that shapes daily life, stress exposure, professional satisfaction, and personal well-being.

In addition to his publishing work, Mason continues to advise healthcare organizations on recruitment strategy, workforce stability, clinician retention, and role-environment alignment — areas that increasingly determine whether healthcare systems can maintain safe staffing levels and consistent patient care quality. His perspective bridges both sides of the hiring equation: the institutional need for stable clinical teams and the individual clinician's need for sustainable career fit.

Mason's writing is known for translating complex workforce realities into practical, real-world guidance. Rather than focusing only on job descriptions or education pathways, his books explore what healthcare roles actually feel like day to day — the pace, decision pressure, collaboration demands, documentation load, emotional intensity, and long-term lifestyle implications that rarely appear in traditional career guides. His goal is simple: help readers **find their fit before they commit**, reducing burnout, turnover, and career regret across the healthcare profession.

Through the **What Color Are Your Scrubs?** flagship career guide and the growing ScrubTales™ series, Mason's work now supports students, career changers, clinicians, educators, and healthcare leaders who want clearer insight into how identity, environment, and role structure intersect to shape career sustainability. His mission is to make alignment a visible part of healthcare career decision-making so that capable people not only enter the profession — but remain in it with purpose, resilience, and long-term fulfillment.

Mason lives and works in the United States and continues to collaborate with healthcare leaders, educators, and clinicians who believe that the future of healthcare depends not only on training more professionals, but on helping them land in roles where they truly belong.

**StaySm:)in'!**

# Also by Mason Maison™ Publishing

**What Color Are Your Scrubs?**

A comprehensive healthcare career guide exploring more than 340 clinical and non-clinical healthcare careers, designed to help readers understand role fit, identity alignment, long-term sustainability, and the real-world emotional and operational demands of modern healthcare work. This flagship volume introduces Mason's alignment-first decision framework and serves as the foundation for the broader ScrubTales™ career exploration ecosystem.

**ScrubTales™ — Real-World Career Guides for Future Healthcare Professionals**

The ScrubTales™ series provides immersive, specialty-focused career exploration books designed to help students, career changers, and early-career clinicians understand what healthcare roles actually feel like in daily practice. Each volume combines cinematic day-in-the-life experiences, hiring and career-navigation systems, financial and workload realities, alignment tools, and practical decision frameworks to help readers evaluate whether a specific healthcare pathway truly fits their personality, pace preferences, and long-term career goals.

**Available and Forthcoming ScrubTales™ Titles Include:**

Nurse Practitioner

Physician Assistant

Registered Nurse

Surgical Technologist

Diagnostic Medical Sonographer

Respiratory Therapist

Clinical Pharmacist

Physical Therapist

Medical Laboratory Scientist

Radiologic Technologist

Licensed Practical Nurse

Medical Assistant

Occupational Therapist

Dental Assistant

Medical and Health Services Manager

Physical Therapist Assistant

Speech-Language Pathologist

Medical Records Specialist

Home Health and Personal Care Aide

Certified Nursing Assistant

Additional ScrubTales™ titles are released regularly as part of Mason Maison™ Publishing's mission to help healthcare professionals **find their fit before they commit**, strengthening long-term workforce stability and career sustainability across the healthcare field.

Made in United States
Orlando, FL
05 November 2026

90231079R00184